*Continued on last page*

# MANUAL *of*
# Nursing
# Diagnosis

## TWELFTH EDITION

*Including all diagnostic categories approved by the
North American Nursing Diagnosis Association*

Marjory Gordon, PhD, RN, FAAN
Professor Emeritus
Cornell School of Nursing
Boston College
Chestnut Hill, Massachusetts

JONES AND BARTLETT PUBLISHERS
*Sudbury, Massachusetts*
BOSTON    TORONTO    LONDON    SINGAPORE

*World Headquarters*
Jones and Bartlett Publishers
40 Tall Pine Drive
Sudbury, MA 01776
978-443-5000
info@jbpub.com
www.jbpub.com

Jones and Bartlett Publishers Canada
6339 Ormindale Way
Mississauga, Ontario L5V 1J2
Canada

Jones and Bartlett Publishers International
Barb House, Barb Mews
London W6 7PA
United Kingdom

Jones and Bartlett's books and products are available through most bookstores
and online booksellers. To contact Jones and Bartlett Publishers directly,
call 800-832-0034, fax 978-443-8000, or visit our website www.jbpub.com.

Substantial discounts on bulk quantities of Jones and Bartlett's publica-
tions are available to corporations, professional associations, and other
qualified organizations. For details and specific discount information,
contact the special sales department at Jones and Bartlett via the above
contact information or send an email to specialsales@jbpub.com.

ISBN: 978-0-7637-7185-0
ISSN: 0748-920X

**Production Credits**
Publisher: Kevin Sullivan
Acquisitions Editor: Emily Ekle
Acquisitions Editor: Amy Sibley
Associate Editor: Patricia Donnelly
Editorial Assistant: Rachel Shuster
Senior Production Editor: Carolyn F. Rogers
Senior Marketing Manager: Barb Bartoszek
V.P., Manufacturing and Inventory Control: Therese Connell
Composition: Graphic World
Cover Design: Scott Moden
Printing and Binding: Courier Westford
Cover Printing: Courier Westford

6048

Printed in the United States of America
13 12 11 10 09   10 9 8 7 6 5 4 3 2 1

# Contents

# Preface

Healthcare delivery is moving quickly toward electronic records for documentation of patient care in hospitals and the community. This requires that care providers record clinical data and their clinical judgments in a clear, concise manner. As with the previous 11 editions, the twelfth edition of the *Manual of Nursing Diagnosis* presents terminology in a way that encourages making diagnostic judgments with clarity and accuracy. Diagnoses and outcomes are organized using 11 health patterns. This is a functional framework, applicable to all clinical specialties and acuity levels. High-risk groups for each diagnosis are identified which increases sensitivity to cues during assessment. Diagnostic (critical) cues are listed which contribute to accuracy in making diagnostic judgments. In addition, outcomes that represent the resolution of nursing diagnoses are included in this twelfth edition.

The inclusion of outcomes encourages nurses to think of the resolution of a condition at the time a diagnosis is made. This is an important factor in the selection of interventions to individualize the delivery of nursing care.

Not all outcomes stated in the manual can be achieved in one care setting or in a short period of time. It may be necessary also to project outcomes that represent steps toward resolution of the condition. This is an aspect of individualizing care.

This manual has proved to be useful to students and clinicians since the first edition in 1982. Diagnoses and assessment categories continue to be organized in the functional health patterns framework. This framework provides a way of assessing health and health management that leads to a holistic approach to nursing care.

The addition of nursing outcomes in this edition should facilitate outcome projection. In turn, the early identification of outcomes will encourage identifying interventions that directly influence outcome achievement. Effective and efficient care, as well as cost saving, will result.

*Marjory Gordon*

## ACKNOWLEDGMENTS

The *Nursing Outcome Classification* influenced the selection of outcomes for many diagnoses. This publication should be consulted for rating scales and more detailed content (see reference on page xvi).

# Use of the Manual

A diagnostic manual can serve many purposes. For students, it is a quick reference during clinical practice, a useful guide in class or clinical conference, and a necessity for doing homework. For expert diagnosticians, it is a clinical reference, a research tool, a teaching or management resource, and a stimulus for ideas. For both learners and experts, it is a much-used companion.

This manual contains the most up-to-date diagnostic categories contained in the NANDA International, Diagnostic Taxonomy. This taxonomy is endorsed by the American Nurses Association and is included in the International Classification for Nursing Practice[1] and Standard Nomenclature of Medicine (SNOMED). Diagnostic terms, definitions of terms, defining characteristics (risk factors for high-risk diagnoses) are included, as are etiological or related factors and high-risk populations for actual diagnoses. One or more outcomes representing resolution of the problem are included for each diagnosis.

The manual supports clinical judgment and decision making in nine major ways:

**Access to nursing diagnoses.** It is a quick reference to terms used in formulating a diagnostic statement and an outcome(s) that describes resolution.

**Use of diagnostic terms.** Each nursing diagnosis term in the manual describes a condition of concern to nurses. The diagnostic term stands for a concept that explains the meaning of a set of cues. As with any terms in a language, each has a standard definition and characteristics.

It is the speaker or writer's responsibility to use the terms correctly. Internationally, nurses are working toward a uniform nursing language and an international classification system of nursing diagnoses.

**Criteria for diagnostic judgments.** When nursing or other research is available, diagnostic cues are specified. In conjunction with supporting data, these are used as criteria for making a diagnosis.

**Functional health pattern assessment guidelines.** Data to diagnosis—guides are included for linking assessment and diagnosis using functional health patterns and diagnostic groupings in the index. In many instances, the client's problem can be formulated by using one diagnostic category to describe the problem and another category from the same, or a different, functional pattern area to describe etiological factors. Risk factors may be in multiple pattern areas.

**High-risk populations.** Some of the conditions described by nursing diagnoses are prevalent in certain groups of people in certain situations or having particular experiences or treatments. High-risk populations of clients/persons are listed in the manual for some diagnoses in which incidence is fairly well established.

**Diagnosis-specific treatment.** The format for developing diagnosis-specific treatment plans is outlined.

**Documentation.** Format, guidelines, and examples of documentation are provided.

**Outcomes.** Outcomes are specified for each diagnosis.

**Special notes.** Pages are included for special notes following each pattern area. The use of this manual for each of these purposes is discussed later here.

# USE OF THE MANUAL

## ACCESS TO NURSING DIAGNOSES

Different situations require different ways of accessing nursing diagnoses. The manual can accommodate the following needs:

> To find a diagnostic category to describe a cluster of signs and symptoms within a functional pattern area, use the Diagnostic Categories on pages xix to xxvi. Diagnoses are grouped by functional patterns. Each diagnosis is clearly presented on its own page.

> When a diagnostic category label is known but you need to check the definition, diagnostic or supporting cues, or etiological/related factors, use the alphabetical index to look up the page number. The alphabetical index serves as a dictionary of diagnostic terms (pages 465 to 482 and inside covers).

> If you wish to scan all the diagnostic categories within a particular functional pattern area, use the contents on pages xix to xxvi as an index to the pattern.

> For research on NANDA-accepted diagnostic categories, use diagnostic categories in *NANDA Nursing Diagnoses: Definitions and Classification, 2009–2011.*[2]

### Use of Diagnostic Terms

The diagnostic categories contained in this manual are concepts used in thinking. They represent a language for communicating professional nurses' diagnostic judgments about actual or potential health problems and health-related conditions. A useful nursing diagnosis statement consists of terms describing (1) the problem or condition and (2) the primary etiological or related factor(s) contributing to the problem or condition that is the focus of nursing treatment.

Many types of judgments are made in practice, but the term nursing diagnosis is reserved for client conditions that "nurses by virtue of their education and experience are capable and licensed to treat."[3] NANDA International's definition of a nursing diagnosis further clarifies the term:

> A nursing diagnosis is a clinical judgment about an individual, family, or community response to actual or potential health problems/life processes which provides the basis for definitive therapy toward achievement of outcomes for which the nurse is accountable.[2]

This builds on a definition based on Shoemaker's research that integrates nursing diagnosis into nursing process:

> Nursing diagnosis is a clinical judgment about an individual, family, or community that is derived through a deliberate, systematic process of data collection and analysis. It provides the basis for prescriptions for definitive therapy for which the nurse is accountable. It is expressed concisely and includes the etiology of the condition when known.[4]

Nursing diagnoses are primarily resolved by nursing care methods, and nurses assume accountability in practice for treatment outcomes. If a diagnosis does not meet these criteria, a notation to refer the problem for medical evaluation will be found on the page containing the diagnosis. An additional characteristic that distinguishes nursing diagnoses is that professional nurses assume responsibility for research on the conditions.

Nurses view the diagnostic categories in this manual from various conceptual perspectives. Depending on the model of nursing used to guide the nursing process and practice, diagnoses may be viewed as self-care agency deficits, ineffective adaptations, human response patterns, needs, or simply dysfunctional health patterns. There is no consensus on the conceptual focus of nursing and thus no consensus on the focus of nursing diagnosis.

Users of the manual should recognize that nursing diagnoses are in the process of development, especially the 30 diagnoses in this manual that are formally under development. Diagnostic categories require conceptual work and further clinical study. It is expected that nurses will modify, delete, and add to the currently accepted classifications. Revisions will occur as diagnoses are used (1) to organize assessment data, (2) as a basis for care planning, and (3) as a focus for nursing documentation. Nurses are encouraged to submit refinements of diagnoses to NANDA International. Diagnoses are reviewed at various levels of development, from just a label and definition to being supported by clinical research. Descriptions of these levels and the process for submission and review can be obtained on the NANDA International Web site.

All diagnostic categories contain the following components: diagnostic category label, definition, defining characteristics (diagnostic and supporting cues), and for actual problems, etiological or related factors. Risk conditions or potential problems have risk factors instead of defining characteristics and etiological factors. Healthy states or processes have factors supporting the patient's desire for health enhancement, rather than etiological/related factors.

Defining characteristics and risk factors are the observations used to make a diagnostic judgment about the presence or absence of a condition. In the manual, defining characteristics are presented as (1) diagnostic cues and (2) supporting cues. Current research evidence suggests that diagnostic cues are the most valid and reliable indicators for diagnosing the condition. Supporting cues used in conjunction with diagnostic cues increase psychological confidence in diagnostic judgments. These cues generally capture variations in behavior across populations and situations. Supporting cues are not specific to one diagnosis; during assessment, they may suggest a few diagnoses. Usually confidence in a diagnostic judgment is attained with the use of the diagnostic cues and some supporting data.

Recommendations of diagnostic and supporting cues in this manual are based on (1) review of research on nursing diagnoses published in NANDA International conference proceedings and in the *International Journal of Nursing Terminologies and Classification;* (2) the author's pooled research data from national studies using 1,100 experts in critical care, rehabilitation, and home care nursing; (3) literature from other disciplines and nursing textbooks when research was minimal or absent; and (4) the author's judgment and logical analysis in the context of diagnostic reasoning and parsimony. For example, if tissue destruction and traumatized tissue are listed, parsimony dictates that the cue, broken skin, is redundant. In a few cases in which diagnoses were not specific (broad taxonomic categories), no recommendation was made. Risk factors may vary with the client population, and insufficient research exists on various populations.

Meta-analyses, integrated research reviews of each diagnosis, concept analysis, and further analyses of data will serve to test the usability of these criteria and the validity of the ratings and diagnostic cues. Nursing research is insufficient for many diagnoses, and in many cases, no replications of large studies exist. In particular, there are minimal studies on possible differences among age and cultural groups. These factors should be kept in mind when using the diagnostic and supporting cues.

The diagnostic cues are used to determine whether the condition described by the diagnosis is present or not. Also, these cues can be used for differential diagnosis among conditions and, most importantly, to justify a diagnostic judgment. For diagnoses that describe a subjective state, diagnostic cues need to include both observation and a verbal report.

Use the nursing diagnoses in the manual as a dictionary of terms and concepts. Clinical experience has demonstrated that the assessment database and the judgment of the nurse determine whether a diagnostic category is used as a probable cause (etiological or related factor) or to describe a problem in the diagnostic statement. For some diagnoses, a footnote is inserted to suggest that the diagnosis is frequently the focus for intervention (i.e., frequently used as an etiological/related factor). In these cases, it describes the probable cause of a problem. Further assessment can reveal the problem.

## FUNCTIONAL HEALTH PATTERN ASSESSMENT: DATA TO DIAGNOSIS

The manual contains an assessment format and diagnostic groupings that facilitate the move from data to diagnosis. Both employ the functional health patterns as a nursing perspective on individual, family, and community health care. It is possible that cognitive strain and diagnostic errors can be reduced if there is consistency between organization of assessment data and grouping of diagnostic categories. For example, if data on the client's elimination pattern can be compared with defining characteristics of diagnoses in the elimination pattern, less effort is required than if the database is unorganized and the very large number of diagnoses is merely alphabetized. The following are guidelines for use of the manual in the diagnostic phase of nursing process:

1. Use the manual both to learn the 11 functional health patterns and to study the diagnostic categories commonly occurring in your practice area. Functional patterns are an easily learned nursing model for assessment. Review the diagram on Components of Nursing Process, pages 40–41 to place nursing diagnosis in the context of nursing process and clinical judgment.

2. Use the assessment guidelines (pages 10–34) that are based on the functional health pattern areas (pages 2–5) to collect and organize a nursing history and examination of adults (pages 11–15), adults in critical care (pages 31–34), infants and young children (pages 16–21), families (pages 21–25), or communiti-es (pages 25–31). Also contained in the manual is a bibliography of

articles on the use of functional health patterns in clinical activities (pages 5–8).

3. If assessment reveals a dysfunctional pattern but the name escapes you, check the diagnoses listed under the pattern (Diagnostic Categories, pages 57–438) for terminology to label the condition. Use the defining characteristics listed with each diagnosis to validate your judgment. Etiological or risk factors listed with each diagnosis may suggest possible reasons for the problem or risk state.

4. For a quick reference before documenting a problem, use either the Diagnostic Categories (pages xix–xxvi), the alphabetical index (pages 465–482 and inside covers), or the quick reference for pages containing diagnoses grouped by the health patterns (outside back cover). Turn to the page corresponding to the possible diagnostic label. Check that the observed signs and symptoms correspond to the defining characteristics of the diagnostic category, particularly the suggested diagnostic cues.

## HIGH-RISK POPULATIONS

Statistics suggest that some conditions described by nursing diagnoses are prevalent in certain groups of people, in certain situations, or during certain experiences or treatments. For example, the population of persons with a stroke and impaired bed mobility is at high risk for pressure ulcer, and older persons living alone with reduced social contacts are prone to depression. The base rate of occurrence is high. Knowing this, clinicians are sensitive to cues during assessment (but exercise caution that statistical incidence of a condition does not affect judgment more than clinical data). Early case finding is due in part to a sensitivity to cues.

In the manual, high-risk populations are listed for some diagnoses in which incidence is fairly well established. Use this information as a basis for raising the possibility that a condition may be present when doing an assessment. Add your own observations to the notes pages that follow each pattern area.

## DIAGNOSIS-SPECIFIC TREATMENT/INTERVENTION

A nursing diagnosis is used as a basis for projecting outcomes, planning interventions, and evaluating outcome attainment. The problem statement is the basis for outcome projection, that is, the identification of behaviors that signify resolution of the problem. These projected outcomes are then used to document progress toward outcome attainment and to evaluate resolution of the problem.

The etiological factor(s) is the focus for designing interventions that will reduce or eliminate the factors contributing to the problem. Outcome attainment is the measure of effectiveness of the intervention. In the case of a potential or high-risk problem, reduction or elimination of risk factors is the desired outcome.

## DOCUMENTATION

Documentation may be carried out in various ways that will be discussed. These include paper, worksheets, and electronic patient records. The Problem-Oriented Recording Format Guidelines and Checkpoints (pages 45–47) will be useful in ensuring consistency between the nursing diagnosis, the projected outcome, and the intervention plan. An example is provided (pages 47–55).

Documentation is important for statistical purposes. Currently, a nursing minimum data set is being studied in a number of countries. This requires documentation of nursing diagnoses, interventions, and outcomes. The nursing minimum data set[5] also includes an acuity factor.

## OUTCOMES

Outcomes are specified for the resolution of each diagnosis. The Nursing Outcomes Classification[6] is used for outcome categories. Each diagnosis has the outcome label and definition describing resolution of the diagnosis. This reference should be consulted for rating scales. For some diagnoses, it may be necessary to use outcomes that specify *steps to resolution. The projected outcome should always be considered when making decisions about nursing interventions.* It specifies the health state to be achieved. The probable cause described by the etiological factor(s) guides specification of time to resolution. The Nursing Interventions Classification is a useful resource for intervention categories and methods.[7]

## SPECIAL NOTES

It is important to learn from practice, rather than just practicing! One of the ways to continue learning is to develop the habit of reflecting on insights and new information, creative interventions, or cost-effective methods. Pages after each pattern area labeled "notes" are valuable for recording clinical information related to each diagnosis such as important additional cues or etiological factors that have been observed, factors related to a specific population of clients, and interventions that are successful in reaching projected outcomes.

## REFERENCES

1. International Council of Nurses. *Nursing's Next Advance: Classification for Nursing Practice.* Geneva, Switzerland: International Council of Nurses; 1994.
2. NANDA International. *Nursing Diagnoses: Definitions and Classification, 2009–2011.* Ames, IA: Wiley-Blackwell; 2009.
3. Gordon M. Nursing diagnosis and the diagnostic process. *Am J Nurs.* 1976;76:1276-1300.
4. Shoemaker J. Essential features of a nursing diagnosis. In Kim MJ, McFarland GK, McLane AM, eds. *Classification of Nursing Diagnoses: Proceedings of the Fifth National Conference.* St. Louis: Mosby; 1984.
5. Werley H, Lang N. *Identification of the Nursing Minimum Data Set.* New York: Springer; 1988.
6. Moorehead S, Johnson M, Maas M, Swanson E. *Nursing Outcome Classification (NOC).* St. Louis: Mosby-Elsevier; 2007.
7. Bulechek GM, Butcher H, McCloskey J. *Nursing Interventions Classification (NIC).* St. Louis: Mosby-Elsevier; 2009.

# Notice

The authors, editor, and publisher have made every effort
to provide accurate information; however, they are not
responsible for errors and omissions or for any outcomes
related to the use of the contents of this book and take no
responsibility for the use of the products described. Research,
clinical practice, and government regulations often change
the accepted standard in this field. In the clinical setting, the
healthcare provider or reader is responsible for determining
the appropriate usage of nursing process and its terminology.

# Diagnostic Categories

Boldface type indicates diagnoses currently accepted by NANDA International (North American Nursing Diagnosis Association). Others are diagnoses developed by the author, not yet reviewed by this association, but are found to be useful in clinical practice. See inside front and back covers for diagnoses arranged in alphabetical order.

## HEALTH PERCEPTION–HEALTH MANAGEMENT PATTERN

# DIAGNOSTIC CATEGORIES

## NUTRITIONAL–METABOLIC PATTERN

## DIAGNOSTIC CATEGORIES

# DIAGNOSTIC CATEGORIES

# DIAGNOSTIC CATEGORIES

## DIAGNOSTIC CATEGORIES

## SELF-PERCEPTION–SELF-CONCEPT PATTERN

# DIAGNOSTIC CATEGORIES

## ROLE–RELATIONSHIP PATTERN

## SEXUALITY–REPRODUCTIVE PATTERN

## DIAGNOSTIC CATEGORIES

# Functional Health
# Patterns Typology

# FUNCTIONAL HEALTH PATTERNS TYPOLOGY

This section contains a typology of health patterns and their definitions that are used for organizing assessment and grouping nursing diagnoses.

## TYPOLOGY

A client's functional health patterns (individuals, families, or communities) evolve from a client–environment interaction. Each pattern is an expression of biopsychosocial integration; thus, no one pattern can be understood without knowledge of the other patterns.

Functional patterns are influenced by biological, developmental, cultural, social, and spiritual factors. A functional pattern represents a healthy set of behaviors. Dysfunctional health patterns (described by nursing diagnoses) may occur with disease; dysfunctional health patterns may also lead to disease.

The judgment of whether a pattern is functional or dysfunctional is made by comparing assessment data to one or more of the following:

1. **INDIVIDUAL BASELINES**

2. **ESTABLISHED NORMS FOR AGE GROUPS**

3. **CULTURAL, SOCIAL, OR OTHER NORMS**

A particular pattern has to be evaluated in the context of other patterns and its contribution to optimal function of the client. The definitions of the health patterns are as follows.

## 1  HEALTH-PERCEPTION–HEALTH-MANAGEMENT PATTERN

Describes the client's perceived pattern of health and well-being and how health is managed. This includes the individual's perception of health status and its relevance to current activities and future planning. Also included is the individual's health-risk management and general healthcare behavior, such as safety practices and adherence to mental and physical health promotion activities, medical or nursing prescriptions, and follow-up care.

## 2 NUTRITIONAL–METABOLIC PATTERN

Describes the pattern of food and fluid consumption relative to metabolic need and pattern indicators of local nutrient supply. This includes the individual's patterns of food and fluid consumption: daily eating times, the types and quantity of food and fluids consumed, particular food preferences, and the use of nutrient or vitamin supplements. It describes breastfeeding and infant feeding patterns and includes reports of any skin lesions, ability to heal, and measures of body temperature, height, and weight. General appearance of well-being and the condition of skin, hair, nails, mucous membranes, and teeth are also included.

## 3 ELIMINATION PATTERN

Describes patterns of excretory function (bowel, bladder, and skin) and includes the individual's perceived regularity of excretory function, the use of routines or laxatives for bowel elimination, and any changes or disturbances in time pattern, mode of excretion, quality, or quantity of elimination. Also included are any devices used to control excretion.

## 4 ACTIVITY–EXERCISE PATTERN

Describes pattern of exercise, activity, leisure, and recreation and includes activities of daily living requiring energy expenditure, such as hygiene, cooking, shopping, eating, working, and home maintenance. Also included are the type, quantity, and quality of exercise, including sports, that describe the typical pattern for the individual. Leisure patterns are also included and describe the activities the client undertakes as recreation either with a group or as an individual. Emphasis is on the activities of high importance or significance and any limitations. Factors that interfere with desired or expected activities for the individual (such as neuromuscular deficits and compensations, dyspnea, angina, or muscle cramping on exertion and cardiac/pulmonary classification, if appropriate) are also included.

## 5 SLEEP–REST PATTERN

Describes patterns of sleep, rest, and relaxation and includes patterns of sleep and rest/relaxation periods during the 24-hour day. Includes perception of the quality and quantity of sleep and rest, perception of energy level after sleep, and any sleep disturbances, as well as aids to sleep such as medications or nighttime routines that the individual uses.

## 6 COGNITIVE–PERCEPTUAL PATTERN

Describes sensory-perceptual and cognitive pattern. Includes the adequacy of sensory modes, such as vision, hearing, taste, touch, and smell and the compensation or prostheses currently used. Reports of pain perception and how pain is managed are included. Also included are cognitive functional abilities such as language, memory, judgment, and decision making.

## 7 SELF-PERCEPTION–SELF-CONCEPT PATTERN

Describes the self-concept pattern and perceptions of mood state. Includes the individual's attitudes about self, perception of abilities (cognitive, affective, or physical), body image, identity, general sense of worth, and general emotional pattern. Body posture and movement, eye contact, voice, and speech pattern are included.

## 8 ROLE–RELATIONSHIP PATTERN

Describes pattern of role engagements and relationships. It includes the individual's perception of the major roles and responsibilities in current life situation. Satisfaction or disturbances in family, work, or social relationships and responsibilities related to these roles are included.

## 9   SEXUALITY–REPRODUCTIVE PATTERN

Describes patterns of satisfaction or dissatisfaction with sexuality and the reproductive pattern. It includes the individual's perceived satisfaction or reports of disturbances in his or her sexuality. Included also is the female's reproductive stage (premenopause or postmenopause) and any perceived problems.

## 10   COPING–STRESS-TOLERANCE PATTERN

Describes the general coping pattern and effectiveness of the pattern in terms of stress tolerance. It includes the individual's reserve or capacity to resist challenge to self-integrity, modes of handling stress, family or other support systems, and perceived ability to manage stressful situations.

## 11   VALUE-BELIEF PATTERN

Describes patterns of values, goals, or beliefs (including spiritual) that guide choices or decisions. It includes what is perceived as important in life, quality of life, and any perceived conflicts in values, beliefs, or expectations that are health related.

### BIBLIOGRAPHY

The following references describe functional health patterns, suggested uses of the patterns, and reports of clinical use and research.

Beyea S, Matzo M. Assessing elders using the functional health pattern assessment model. *Nurse Educ*. 1989;14:32–37.

Bryant SO, Kopeski LM. Psychiatric nursing assessment of the eating disorder client. *Top Clin Nurs*. 1986;8:57–66.

Burns C. Development and content validity testing of a comprehensive classification of diagnoses for pediatric nurse practitioners. *Nurs Diagn*. 1991;2:93–104.

Burns C. *Development and Field Testing of a Classification of Diagnoses for Use by Pediatric Nurse Practitioners* [dissertation]. Eugene, OR: University of Oregon; 1989.

# FUNCTIONAL HEALTH PATTERNS TYPOLOGY

Coler MS, Vincent KG. Coded nursing diagnoses on axes: a prioritized, computer–ready diagnostic system for psychiatric–mental health nurses. *Arch Psychiatr Nurs.* 1987;1:125–131.

Collard A, Jones DA, Fitzmaurice J. *Nursing Diagnoses in Ambulatory Care.* In McLane A, ed. Classification of Nursing Diagnoses: Proceedings of the Seventh Conference. St. Louis, MO: Mosby; 1987.

Corrigan JO. Functional health pattern assessment in the emergency department. *J Emerg Nurs.* 1986;12:163–167.

Decker SD, Knight L. Functional health pattern assessment: a seasonal farmworker community. *J Comm Health Nurs.* 1990;7:141–151.

de Hulla M. *Nursing Diagnoses in Relation to Nausea and Vomiting Caused by Chemotherapy.* In Mortensen RA, ed. Proceedings of the First European Conference on Nursing Diagnoses. Copenhagen, Denmark: Danish Institute for Health and Nursing Research; 1995.

Di Blasi M, Savage J. Revitalizing a documentation system. *Rehabil Nurs.* 1992;17:27–29.

Dion P, Fitzmaurice J, Baer C. *Organization of Patient Assessment Data and Nursing Diagnosis.* In McLane A, ed. Classification of Nursing Diagnoses: Proceedings of the Seventh Conference. St. Louis, MO: Mosby; 1987.

Doyer B, Macker N, Radovich H. Functional health patterns: a postanesthesia care unit's approach to identification. *J Post Anesth Nurs.* 1990;5:157–162.

Erdemir F. Utilization of nursing diagnoses by students during a pediatric nursing course in Turkey. *Int J Nurs Terminol Class.* 2003;14:59.

Flanagan J, Jones DA. Patient response to the fast-track experience. *Int J Terminol Class.* 2003;14:42.

Gilmartin ME. Patient and family education. *Clin Chest Med.* 1986;7:619–627.

Gordon M. *Assess Notes: Nursing Assessment and Diagnostic Reasoning.* Philadelphia: F.A. Davis; 2008.

Gordon M. Capturing Patient Problems: Nursing Diagnoses and Functional Health Patterns. In Naming Nursing: Proceedings of the first ACENDIO Ireland/UK Conference in Swansea, Wales, UK. Bern, Switzerland: Verlag-Hans Huber; 2003.

Gordon M. Classification of Nursing Diagnoses: Functional Health Patterns and the NANDA Taxonomy. In Mortensen RA, ed. Proceedings of the First European Conference on Nursing Diagnoses. Copenhagen, Denmark: Danish Institute for Health and Nursing Research; 1995.

Gordon M. *Nursing Diagnosis and Nursing Theory: Expert Nurse 8.* Tokyo, Japan: Shorinsha; 2000.

Gordon M. *Nursing Diagnosis: Process and Application.* St. Louis, MO: Mosby; 1994.

Gordon M. Practice–based data set for a nursing information system. *J Med Syst.* 1985;9:43–55.

Gordon M, Sato S. *Easy to Understand Functional Health Patterns.* Tokyo, Japan: Shorinsha; 1998.

# FUNCTIONAL HEALTH PATTERNS TYPOLOGY

Greenlee KK. Effects of Implementation of an Operational Definition and Guidelines for the Formulation of Nursing Diagnoses in a Critical Care Setting. In Carroll-Johnson R, ed. Classification of Nursing Diagnoses: Proceedings of the Ninth Conference. St. Louis, MO: Mosby; 1991.

Hanna D, Wyman N. Assessment 1 diagnosis 5 care planning: a tool for coordination. *Nurs Manage.* 1989;18:106–109.

Hartman D, Knudson J. Documentation: a nursing data base for initial patient assessment. *Oncol Nurs Forum.* 1991;18:125–130.

Henning M. Comparison of Nursing Diagnostic Statements Using a Functional Health Pattern and Health History/Body Systems Format. In Carroll-Johnson R, ed. Classification of Nursing Diagnoses: Proceedings of the Ninth Conference. St. Louis, MO: Mosby; 1991.

Herberth L, Gosnell DJ. Nursing diagnosis for oncology nursing practice. *Cancer Nurs.* 1987;10:41–51.

Hirschfield-Bartek J, Dow KH. Decreasing documentation time using a patient self-assessment tool. *Oncol Nurs Forum.* 1990;17:251–255.

Hovey JE. Development of a Psychiatric Nursing Assessment Tool Utilizing Functional Health Patterns. In Rantz MJ, LeMone P, eds. Classification of Nursing Diagnoses: Proceedings of the Eleventh Conference. Glendale, CA: CINAHL Information Systems; 1995.

Johannesma JC. Diagnostic Procedures and Nursing Diagnoses for the Elderly. In Mortensen RA, ed. Proceedings of the First European Conference on Nursing Diagnoses. Copenhagen, Denmark: Danish Institute for Health and Nursing Research; 1995.

Johnson M, Maas M, Moorhead S. *Nursing Outcomes Classification (NIC).* St. Louis, MO: Mosby; 2000.

Jones DA. Alternative Conceptualizations of Assessment. In Carroll-Johnson R, Paquette M, eds. Classification of Nursing Diagnoses: Proceedings of the Tenth Conference. Philadelphia: Lippincott; 1994.

Jones DA, Foster FB. Further Development and Testing of a Functional Health Pattern Assessment Screening Tool. In Rantz M, LeMone P, eds. Classification of Nursing Diagnoses: Proceedings of the Thirteenth Conference. Glendale, CA: CINAHL Information Systems; 1999.

Leahy MK. Using Nursing Diagnosis as an Organizing Framework in an Integrated Curriculum. In Jones A, ed. From Theory to Practice: Abstracts of the Second Nursing Theory Congress. Toronto, Ontario: University of Toronto Press; 1988.

Levin RF, Crosley JM. Focused data collection for the generation of nursing diagnoses. *J Nurs Staff Dev.* 1986;4:56–64.

McCourt A, ed. *The Specialty Practice of Rehabilitation Nursing: A Core Curriculum,* 3rd ed. Skokie, IL: Rehabilitation Nursing Foundation; 1993.

McFarland G, Thomas MD. *Psychiatric Mental Health Nursing.* Philadelphia: Lippincott; 1990.

Monninger E, Padgett D, Fleeger MA. Functional Health Pattern Assessment for BSN Students. In Carroll-Johnson R, Paquette M, eds. Classification of

Nursing Diagnoses: Proceedings of the Tenth Conference. Philadelphia, PA: Lippincott; 1994.

Monteiro da Cruz, Dina de Almeida Lopes. Nursing Diagnosis of Patients with Chagas Disease. In Rantz M, LeMone P, eds. Classification of Nursing Diagnoses: Proceedings of the Eleventh Conference. Glendale, CA: CINAHL Information Systems; 1995.

Mumma CM, ed. *Rehabilitation Nursing: Concepts and Practice: A Core Curriculum*, 2nd ed. Skokie, IL: Rehabilitation Nursing Foundation; 1987.

NANDA International. NANDA Nursing Diagnosis Classification, Taxonomy II. In NANDA International Nursing Diagnoses: Definitions and Classification, 2005–2006. Philadelphia: NANDA International; 2005. (Taxonomy domains adapted from Gordon M, Functional Health Patterns Framework.)

Nettle C, Jones N, Pifer P. Community nursing diagnoses. *Commun Health Nurs.* 1989;6:135–145.

O'Connell BO. Does an Assessment Format Influence Diagnostic Outcomes? A Comparison Between Gordon's Functional Health Patterns and a Review of Biological Systems Assessment Formats. In Mortensen RA, ed. Proceedings of the First European Conference on Nursing Diagnoses. Copenhagen, Denmark: Danish Institute for Health and Nursing Research; 1995.

Oud NE. Nursing Diagnoses and Applications in Psychiatric and Mental Nursing. In Mortensen RA, ed. Proceedings of the First European Conference on Nursing Diagnoses. Copenhagen, Denmark: Danish Institute for Health and Nursing Research; 1995.

Phelan C, Finnell MD, Mottla KA. A patient self-assessment tool for cardiac rehabilitation. *Rehabil Nurs.* 1989;14:81, 84–87.

Rantz M, Miller TV. How diagnoses are changing in long-term care. *Am J Nurs.* 1987;87:360–361.

Rossi L. Organizing Data for Nursing Diagnosis Using Functional Health Patterns. In McLane A, ed. Classification of Nursing Diagnoses: Proceedings of the Seventh Conference. St. Louis, MO: Mosby; 1987.

Tompkins ES. In support of the discipline of nursing: a nursing assessment. *Nurs Connect.* 1989;2:21–29.

Volpato MP. Nursing diagnoses in medical-surgical patients. *Int J Nurs Terminol Class.* 2003;14:57.

Ward CR. Proportion of Specific Agreement as a Measure of Intrarater Reliability in the Diagnostic Process. In McLane A, ed. Classification of Nursing Diagnoses: Proceedings of the Seventh Conference. St. Louis, MO: Mosby; 1987.

Westwell J, et al. Health Patterns Assessment: A Form Designed to Allow Psychiatric Nurses to Practice Theoretical Pluralism. In Jones A, ed. From Theory to Practice: Abstracts of the Second Nursing Theory Congress. Toronto, Ontario: University of Toronto Press; 1988.

Woodtli MA, Van Ort S. Nursing diagnoses and functional health patterns in patients receiving external radiation therapy: cancer of the head and neck. *Nurs Diagn.* 1991;2:171–180.

# Functional Health Patterns Assessment Guidelines

## FUNCTIONAL HEALTH PATTERNS ASSESSMENT GUIDELINES

This section contains assessment guidelines based on the health pattern definitions. Functional health patterns provide a format for the admission assessment and a database for nursing diagnoses. There are two phases in assessment: history taking and examination. A nursing history provides a description of a client's functional patterns. The description is from the individual (or parent/guardian), family, or community representative's perspective. It provides subjective data in the form of verbal reports. These reports are elicited by questions that assist clients to tell the history and current status of their health and health management. Observations in the examination phase provide data on pattern indicators and verification of information obtained during history taking. This is referred to as objective data.

The formats for assessment that follow are designed to elicit information in a systematic manner. They are screening formats for the collection of a basic nursing database in any specialty, for any age group, and at any point in the wellness–illness continuum. Questions and examination items tap into areas of all current nursing diagnoses. If data indicate that a problem or potential problem (dysfunctional pattern) may be present, diagnostic hypotheses (nursing diagnoses) should be generated to direct further information collection. This directs the search for the diagnostic or critical characteristics of each possibility.

Nurses practicing in a specialty area may desire in-depth assessments of certain patterns. Both the history (subjective data) and the examination (objective data) can be expanded relative to disease, disability, age, and other client-specific factors. For example, a client's activity–exercise pattern requires an in-depth assessment when the client has a disease that affects this pattern.

Diagnoses are grouped under the same pattern areas as they are in the assessment guidelines and are used to label tentative judgments in a pattern area. As discussed previously, this facilitates the process of moving from assessment data to diagnosis.

# FUNCTIONAL HEALTH PATTERNS ASSESSMENT GUIDELINES

## ADULT ASSESSMENT

### Nursing History

1. **HEALTH-PERCEPTION–HEALTH-MANAGEMENT PATTERN**
   a. How has general health been?
   b. Any colds in the past year? If appropriate, absences from work/school?
   c. Most important things done to keep healthy? Did these things make a difference to health (include family folk remedies, if appropriate)? Breast self-examination? Use cigarettes? Drugs? Ever had a drinking problem? When was your last drink?
   d. Accidents (home, work, driving)? Falls?
   e. In past, easy to find ways to follow suggestions of doctors or nurses?
   f. If appropriate, what do you think caused this illness? Action taken when symptoms perceived? Results of action?
   g. If appropriate, what is important to you while you are here? How can we be most helpful?

2. **NUTRITIONAL–METABOLIC PATTERN**
   a. Typical daily food intake? Describe. Supplements?
   b. Typical daily fluid intake? Describe.
   c. Weight loss/gain? Amount? Height loss/gain? Amount?
   d. Appetite?
   e. Food or eating discomfort? Swallowing? Diet restrictions? If appropriate, breastfeeding? Problems with breastfeeding?
   f. Heal well or poorly?
   g. Skin problems, such as lesions, dryness?
   h. Dental problems?

# FUNCTIONAL HEALTH PATTERNS ASSESSMENT GUIDELINES

## 3. ELIMINATION PATTERN

   a. Bowel elimination pattern? Describe. Frequency?
      Character? Discomfort? Problem in control?
      Laxatives?
   b. Urinary elimination pattern? Describe. Frequency?
      Discomfort? Problem in control?
   c. Excess perspiration? Odor problems?

## 4. ACTIVITY–EXERCISE PATTERN

   a. Sufficient energy for desired/required activities?
   b. Exercise pattern? Type? Regularity?
   c. Spare time (leisure) activities? Child's play activities?
   d. Perceived ability for the following (code level
      according to Functional Levels Code below)

| | | | |
|---|---|---|---|
| Feeding | _____ | Grooming | _____ |
| Bathing | _____ | General mobility | _____ |
| Toileting | _____ | Cooking | _____ |
| Bed mobility | _____ | Home maintenance | _____ |
| Dressing | _____ | Shopping | _____ |

### Functional Levels Code

| | |
|---|---|
| Level 0: | Full self-care |
| Level I: | Requires use of equipment or device |
| Level II: | Requires assistance or supervision of another person |
| Level III: | Requires assistance or supervision of another person and equipment or device |
| Level IV: | Is dependent and does not participate |

## 5. SLEEP–REST PATTERN

   a. Generally rested and ready for daily activities after
      sleep?
   b. Sleep-onset problems? Aids? Dreams (nightmares)?
      Early awakening?
   c. Rest/relaxation periods?

## 6. COGNITIVE–PERCEPTUAL PATTERN

   a. Hearing difficulty? Aid?
   b. Vision? Wear glasses? Last checked?
   c. Any change in memory lately?
   d. Easy/difficult to make decisions?
   e. Easiest way for you to learn things? Any difficulty learning?
   f. Any discomfort? Pain? How do you manage it?

## 7. SELF-PERCEPTION–SELF-CONCEPT PATTERN

   a. How would you describe yourself? Most of the time, do you feel good (not so good) about yourself?
   b. Changes in your body or the things you can do? Are these problematic for you?
   c. Changes in way you feel about yourself or your body (since illness started)?
   d. Find things frequently make you angry? Annoyed? Fearful? Anxious? Depressed? What helps?
   e. Ever feel you lose hope? Not able to control things in life? What helps?

## 8. ROLE–RELATIONSHIP PATTERN

   a. Live alone? Family? Family structure? Draw diagram.
   b. Any family problems you have difficulty handling (nuclear/extended)?
   c. How does the family usually handle problems?
   d. Family depend on you for things? How are you managing?
   e. If appropriate, how do family/others feel about your illness/hospitalization?
   f. If appropriate, problems with children? Difficulty handling?
   g. Belong to social groups? Close friends? Feel lonely (frequency)?

   h. Things generally go well for you at work? School? If appropriate, income sufficient for needs?

   i. Feel part of (or isolated in) neighborhood where living?

## 9. SEXUALITY–REPRODUCTIVE PATTERN

   a. If appropriate to age/situation, sexual relationships satisfying? Changes? Problems?

   b. If appropriate, use of contraceptives? Problems?

   c. For females, when menstruation started? Last menstrual period? Menstrual problems? Para? Gravida?

## 10. COPING–STRESS-TOLERANCE PATTERN

   a. Any big changes in your life in the last year or two? Crisis?

   b. Who's most helpful in talking things over? Available to you now?

   c. Tense a lot of the time? What helps? Use any medicines, drugs, alcohol?

   d. When (if) problems occur in your life, how do you handle them?

   e. Most of the time, is this way(s) successful?

## 11. VALUE–BELIEF PATTERN

   a. Generally get things you want out of life? Important plans for the future?

   b. Religion important in your life? If appropriate, does this help when difficulties arise?

   c. If appropriate, will being here interfere with any religious practices?

## 12. OTHER

   a. Any other things that we have not talked about that you would like to mention?

   b. Questions?

## FUNCTIONAL HEALTH PATTERNS ASSESSMENT GUIDELINES

### SCREENING EXAMINATION FORMAT

Add other pattern indicators to expand the examination as appropriate.

    a. General appearance, grooming, hygiene _____

    b. Oral mucous membranes (color, moistness, lesions) \_\_\_

    c. Teeth: Dentures \_\_\_\_\_ Cavities \_\_\_\_\_ Missing _____

    d. Hears whisper? _____

    e. Reads newsprint? _____ Glasses? _____

    f. Pulse (rate) \_\_\_\_\_ (rhythm) \_\_\_\_\_ (strength) _____

    g. Respiration \_\_\_\_\_ (depth) \_\_\_\_\_ (rhythm) _____

    h. Breath sounds _____ Blood pressure _____

    i. Hand grip _____ Can pick up pencil? _____

    j. Range of motion (joints) Muscle firmness (tone) \_\_\_\_

    k. Skin: Bony prominences _____ Lesions _____
       Color changes _____

    l. Gait \_\_\_\_\_ Posture \_\_\_\_\_ Absent body part \_\_\_\_\_

    m. Demonstrated ability for the following (code for
       level):

| | | |
|---|---|---|
| Feeding _____ | | Grooming _____ |
| Bathing _____ | | General mobility _____ |
| Toileting _____ | | Cooking _____ |
| Bed mobility _____ | | Home maintenance _____ |
| Dressing _____ | | Shopping _____ |

    n. Intravenous, drainage, suction, etc. (specify) _____

    o. Actual weight _____ Reported weight _____

    p. Height _____ Temperature _____

During history and examination:

    q. Orientation _____ Grasp ideas and questions
       (abstract, concrete)? _____

    r. Language spoken; voice and speech pattern _____

    s. Vocabulary level _____

    t. Eye contact \_\_\_\_\_ Attention span (distraction) \_\_\_\_\_

    u. Nervous (5) or relaxed (1) (rate from 1 to 5) _____

    v. Assertive (5) or passive (1) (rate from 1 to 5) _____

    w. Interaction with family member, guardian, other
       (if present) _____

## FUNCTIONAL HEALTH PATTERNS ASSESSMENT GUIDELINES

### INFANT AND YOUNG CHILD ASSESSMENT

When a new infant or child is added to a nurse's caseload, a comprehensive assessment is done to establish a database for developmental assessment and for nursing diagnosis and treatment. Information is needed on (1) the development of each functional pattern and anatomical growth, (2) current health patterns, and (3) family health and the home environment in which the infant or child is developing. Minimally, the admission nursing history and examination has to screen for high-incidence problems. The questions and items listed below can be used as a guide for a comprehensive parent–child health history or used selectively for problem screening.

### NURSING HISTORY

1. **HEALTH-PERCEPTION–HEALTH-MANAGEMENT PATTERN**

Parent's report of
   a. Mother's pregnancy/labor/delivery history (of this infant, of others)?
   b. Infant's health status since birth?
   c. Adherence to routine health checks for the infant/child? Immunizations?
   d. Infections in the infant/child? Child's absences from school?
   e. If appropriate, infant's/child's medical problem, treatment, and prognosis?
   f. If appropriate, actions taken by parents when signs and/or symptoms were perceived?
   g. If appropriate, has it been easy to follow doctor's or nurse's suggestions?
   h. Preventive health practices (e.g., diaper change, utensils, and clothes)?
   i. Do parents smoke? Around children?
   j. Accidents? Frequency?

    k.  Infant's crib toys (safety)? Carrying safety? Car safety?

    l.  Parents' safety practices (e.g., household products and medicines)?

Parents (self)

    a.  Parents'/family's general health status?

## 2. NUTRITIONAL–METABOLIC PATTERN

Parent's report of the infant/child's

    a.  Breast/bottle feeding? Intake (estimated)? Sucking strength?

    b.  Appetite? Feeding discomfort?

    c.  24-Hour intake of nutrients? Supplements?

    d.  Eating behavior? Food preferences? Conflicts over food?

    e.  Birth weight? Current weight?

    f.  Skin problems: rashes, lesions, other?

Parents (self)

    a.  Parent/family's nutritional status? Problems?

## 3. ELIMINATION PATTERN

Parent's report of the infant/child's

    a.  Bowel elimination pattern? Describe. Frequency? Character? Discomfort?

    b.  Diaper changes? Describe routine.

    c.  Urinary elimination pattern? Describe. Number of wet diapers per day? Estimate amount. Stream (strong, dribble)?

    d.  Excess perspiration? Odor?

Parents (self)

    a.  Elimination pattern? Problems?

## 4. ACTIVITY–EXERCISE PATTERN

Parent's report of

    a.  Bathing routine (when, how, where, and what type of soap)?

    b.  Dressing routine (clothing worn, changes inside/outside home)?

    c.  Typical day's activity for the infant/child (e.g., hours spent in crib, being carried, playing; type of toys used)?

    d.  Infant's/child's general activity level? Tolerance?

    e.  Perception of infant's/child's strength (strong or fragile)?

    f.  Child's self-care ability (bathing, feeding, toileting, dressing, grooming)?

Parents (self)

    a.  Activity/exercise/leisure pattern? Child care? Home maintenance?

## 5. SLEEP–REST PATTERN

Parent's report of

    a.  Sleep pattern of the infant/child? Estimated hours?

    b.  Infant/child's restlessness? Nightmares? Nocturia?

    c.  Infant's sleep position? Body movements?

Parents (self)

    a.  Sleep pattern?

## 6. COGNITIVE–PERCEPTUAL PATTERN

Parent's report of

    a.  General responsiveness of the infant/child?

    b.  Infant's response to talking? Noise? Objects? Touch?

    c.  Infant's following of objects with eyes? Response to crib toys?

    d.  Learning (changes noted)? What is being taught to the infant/child?

    e.  Noises/vocalizations? Speech pattern? Words? Sentences?

    f.  Use of stimulation? Talking, games, what else?

    g.  Vision, hearing, touch, kinesthesia of the infant/child?

    h. Child's ability to tell name, time, address, telephone number?

    i. Infant's/child's ability to identify needs (hunger, thirst, pain, discomfort)?

Parents (self)

    a. Problems with vision, hearing, touch, other senses?

    b. Difficulties making decisions? Judgments?

## 7. SELF-PERCEPTION–SELF-CONCEPT PATTERN

Parent's report of

    a. Infant's/child's mood state (irritability)?

    b. Child's sense of worth, identity, competency?

Child's report of

    a. Mood state?

    b. Many/few friends? Liked by others?

    c. Self-perception? Good most of time? Hard to be good?

    d. Ever lonely?

    e. Fears (transient/frequent)?

Parents (self)

    a. General sense of worth, identity, competency?

    b. Self-perception as parents?

## 8. ROLE–RELATIONSHIP PATTERN

Parent's report of

    a. Family/household structure?

    b. Family problems/stressors?

    c. Interactions among family members and infant (or child)?

    d. Infant's/child's response to separation?

    e. Child's dependency?

    f. Child's play pattern?

    g. Child's temper tantrums? Discipline problems? School adjustment?

# FUNCTIONAL HEALTH PATTERNS ASSESSMENT GUIDELINES

Parents (self)
   a. Role engagements? Satisfaction?
   b. Work, social, marital relationships?

## 9. SEXUALITY–REPRODUCTIVE PATTERN

Parent's report of child's
   a. Feeling of maleness/femaleness?
   b. Questions regarding sexuality? How parent responds?
Parents (self)
   a. If applicable, reproductive history?
   b. Sexual satisfaction/problems?

## 10. COPING–STRESS-TOLERANCE PATTERN

Parent's report of
   a. What produces stress in child? Level of stress tolerance?
   b. Child's pattern of handling problems, frustrations, anger?
Parents (self)
   a. Life stressors? Family stress?
   b. Strategies for handling problems? Support systems?

## 11. VALUE–BELIEF PATTERN

Parent's report of
   a. Child's moral development, choice behavior, commitments?
Parents (self)
   a. Things important in life (values, spirituality)? Desires for the future?
   b. If appropriate, perceived impact of disease on goals?

## 12. OTHER

   a. Any other things that we haven't talked about that you'd like to mention? Any questions?

# FUNCTIONAL HEALTH PATTERNS ASSESSMENT GUIDELINES

## SCREENING EXAMINATION FORMAT

a. General appearance of infant/child _____
b. General appearance of parents _____
c. Child's height/weight _____
   Structural growth and development _____
d. Skin color, hydration, rashes, lesions _____
e. If warranted examine: Child's/infant's urine
   and stool _____
f. Reflexes (appropriate to age?) _____
   Blood pressure _____
g. Breathing pattern: rate, rhythm _____
h. Heart sounds: rate, rhythm _____
i. Infant/child: responsiveness, cognitive-perceptual
   development _____
j. Child: eye contact, speech pattern, posturing _____
k. Smiling response (infant) _____
l. Social interaction (child):
   Aggressive/withdrawn? _____
m. Response to vocalizations? Requests? _____

## FAMILY ASSESSMENT

The 11 functional health pattern areas are also applicable
to the assessment of families. Families are the primary
client in community health nursing. In some cases, a family
assessment may be indicated (1) in the care of an infant or
child whose development is influenced by family health patterns or (2) when an adult has certain health problems that
can be influenced by family patterns or can influence these
patterns. The following guidelines provide information on
family functioning.

### 1. HEALTH-PERCEPTION–HEALTH-MANAGEMENT PATTERN

History
a. How has the family's general health been (in last few
   years)?

b. Colds in past year? Absence from work/school?
c. Most important things to keep healthy? Think these make a difference to health (include family folk remedies, if appropriate)?
d. Family members' use of cigarettes, alcohol, drugs?
e. Immunizations? Health care provider? Frequency of checkups?
f. Accidents (home, work, school, driving) (if appropriate, storage of drugs, cleaning products, use of scatter rugs, etc.)?
g. In past, easy to find ways to follow suggestions of doctors, nurses, social workers (if appropriate)?
h. Things important to family's health that I could help with?

Examination

a. General appearance of family members and home.
b. If appropriate, storage of medicines, location of cribs, playpens, stove, scatter rugs, hazards, and other potentially harmful objects.

## 2. NUTRITIONAL–METABOLIC PATTERN

History

a. Typical family meal pattern/food intake? (describe) Supplements (e.g., vitamins, types of snacks)?
b. Typical family fluid intake? Describe. Supplements: type (e.g., fruit juices, soft drinks, coffee)?
c. Appetite? Problems? Dental care (frequency)?
d. Anyone have skin problems? Healing problems?

Examination

a. If opportunity available: refrigerator contents, meal preparation, contents of meal, dining area.

## 3. ELIMINATION PATTERN

History

a. Family use of laxatives, other aids?
b. Problems in waste/garbage disposal?

    c. Pet animals' waste disposal (indoor/outdoor)?

    d. If indicated, problems with flies, roaches, rodents?

Examination

    a. If opportunity available, examine toilet facilities, garbage disposal, pet waste disposal; indicators of risk for flies, roaches, rodents.

### 4. ACTIVITY–EXERCISE PATTERN

History

    a. In general, does family get a lot of exercise or little exercise? Type? Regularity?

    b. Family leisure activities? Active or passive?

    c. Problems in shopping (transportation), cooking, keeping up the house, budgeting for food, clothes, housekeeping, housing costs?

Examination

    a. Pattern of general home maintenance, personal maintenance.

### 5. SLEEP–REST PATTERN

History

    a. Generally, do family members seem to be well rested and ready for school or work?

    b. Sufficient sleeping space and quiet?

    c. Does family find time to relax?

Examination

    a. If opportunity available, observe sleeping space and arrangements.

### 6. COGNITIVE–PERCEPTUAL PATTERN

History

    a. Visual or hearing problems? How managed?

    b. Any big decisions family has had to make? How made?

Examination

    a. If indicated, language spoken at home

    b. Grasp of ideas and questions (abstract or concrete)

    c. Vocabulary level

# FUNCTIONAL HEALTH PATTERNS ASSESSMENT GUIDELINES

## 7. SELF-PERCEPTION–SELF-CONCEPT PATTERN

History
    a. Most of time family feels good (not so good) about themselves as a family?
    b. General mood of family? Happy? Anxious? Depressed? What helps family mood?

Examination
    a. General mood state: relaxed (1) or nervous (5); rate from 1 to 5.
    b. Members generally passive (1) or assertive (5); rate from 1 to 5.

## 8. ROLE–RELATIONSHIP PATTERN

History
    a. Family (or household) members' age and family structure? Draw diagram.
    b. Any family problems that are difficult to handle (nuclear/extended)? Child rearing? If appropriate, spouse ever get rough with you? Children?
    c. Relationships good (not so good) among family members? Siblings?
    d. If appropriate, income sufficient for needs?
    e. Feel part of (or isolated from) community? Neighbors?

Examination
    a. Interaction among family members (if present).
    b. Observed family leadership roles.

## 9. SEXUALITY–REPRODUCTIVE PATTERN

History
    a. If appropriate (sexual partner within household or situation), sexual relations satisfying? Changes? Problems?
    b. Use of family planning? Contraceptives? Problems?

    c. If appropriate (to age of children), feel comfortable in explaining/discussing sexual subjects?

Examination

    a. None

## 10. COPING–STRESS-TOLERANCE PATTERN

History

    a. Any big changes within family in last few years?

    b. Family tense or relaxed most of time? When tense, what helps? Anyone use medicines, drugs, alcohol to decrease tension? Support each other?

    c. When family problems arise, how handled?

    d. Most of the time is this way(s) successful?

Examination

    a. None

## 11. VALUE–BELIEF PATTERN

History

    a. Generally, family get things they want out of life?

    b. Important things for the future?

    c. Any "rules" in the family that everyone believes are important?

    d. Religion important in family? Does this help when difficulties arise?

Examination

    a. None

## COMMUNITY ASSESSMENT*

Communities develop health patterns. In some practice settings, the community is the primary client. In other cases, an individual client or a family may have or be predisposed to

*Community assessment items are adapted from Gikow F, Kucharski P. Functional health pattern assessment of a community. Paper presented at: American Public Health Association, 112th annual meeting; November 13, 1984; Anaheim, Calif. Gikow and Kucharski used the functional assessment to evaluate health-related needs of a community served by their agency.

certain problems that require an assessment of certain community patterns. The following are guidelines for a comprehensive community assessment, but particular community patterns may be relevant to care of an individual or family. In addition, if a community health nurse or agency does not wish to obtain an in-depth study of a community, screening of functional patterns is possible by selecting items from the examination sections.

## 1. HEALTH-PERCEPTION–HEALTH-MANAGEMENT PATTERN

History (Community Representatives)

a. In general, what is the health/wellness level of the population on a scale of 1 to 5, with 5 being high? Any major health problems?

b. Any strong cultural patterns influencing health practices?

c. Do people feel they have access to health services?

d. Is there demand for any particular health services or prevention programs?

e. Do people feel fire, police, safety programs are sufficient?

Examination (Community Records)

a. Morbidity, mortality, disability rates (by age group, if appropriate).

b. Accident rates (by district, if appropriate).

c. Currently operating health facilities (types).

d. Ongoing health promotion/prevention programs, utilization rates.

e. Ratios of health professionals to population.

f. Laws regarding drinking age.

g. Arrest statistics for drug use and/or drunk driving by age group.

## 2. NUTRITIONAL-METABOLIC PATTERN

History (Community Representatives)

a. In general, do most people seem well nourished? Children? Older persons?

b. Food supplement programs? Food stamps: rate of use?

c. Is cost of foods reasonable in this area relative to income?

d. Are stores accessible for most? Meals on Wheels available?

e. Water supply and quality? Testing services (if most have own wells)? If appropriate, water usage cost? Any drought restrictions?

f. Any concern that community growth will exceed good water supply?

g. Are heating/cooling costs manageable for most? Programs?

Examination

a. General appearance (nutrition, teeth, clothing appropriate for climate). Children? Adults? Older persons?

b. Food purchases (observations at food store checkout counters).

c. "Junk" food (e.g., machines in schools).

## 3. ELIMINATION PATTERN

History (Community Representatives)

a. Major kinds of wastes (e.g., industrial, sewage)? Disposal systems? Recycling programs? Any problems perceived by community?

b. Pest control? Food service inspection (e.g., restaurants, street vendors)?

Examination (Community Records)

a. Communicable disease statistics

b. Air pollution statistics

## 4. ACTIVITY-EXERCISE PATTERN

History (Community Representatives)

    a. How do people find the transportation here? To work? For recreation? To health care?

    b. Do people (seniors, others) have/use community centers? Recreation facilities for children? Adults? Seniors?

    c. Is housing adequate (availability, cost)? Public housing?

Examination

    a. Recreation/cultural programs

    b. Assistance for the disabled

    c. Residential centers, nursing homes, rehabilitation facilities relative to population needs

    d. External maintenance of homes, yards, apartment houses

    e. General activity level (e.g., bustling, quiet)

## 5. SLEEP–REST PATTERN

History (Community Representatives)

    a. Generally quiet at night in most neighborhoods?

    b. Usual business hours? Are industries active around the clock?

Examination

    a. Activity/noise levels in business district, residential area

## 6. COGNITIVE–PERCEPTUAL PATTERN

History

    a. Do most groups speak English? Bilingual?

    b. Educational level of population?

    c. Schools seen as good or need improving? Adult education desired or available?

    d. Types of problems that require community decisions? Decision-making process? What is best way to get things done/changed in community?

# FUNCTIONAL HEALTH PATTERNS ASSESSMENT GUIDELINES

Examination
- a. School facilities, dropout rate.
- b. Community government structure, decision-making lines.

## 7. SELF-PERCEPTION–SELF-CONCEPT PATTERN

History (Community Representatives)
- a. Good community to live in? Status going up, down, or staying about the same?
- b. Old community? Fairly new?
- c. Does any age group predominate?
- d. People's mood, in general: Enjoying life? Stressed? Feeling "down"?
- e. People generally have the kinds of abilities needed in this community?
- f. Community/neighborhood functions? Parades?

Examination
- a. Racial, ethnic mix (if appropriate).
- b. Socioeconomic level.
- c. General observations of mood.

## 8. ROLE–RELATIONSHIP PATTERN

History (Community Representatives)
- a. Do people seem to get along well together here? Places where people tend to go to socialize?
- b. Do people feel they are heard by the government? High or low participation in meetings?
- c. Enough work/jobs for everybody? Are wages good/fair? Do people seem to like the type of work available (happy in their jobs or feel job stress)?
- d. Any problems with riots, violence in the neighborhoods? Family violence? Problems with child/spouse/older person abuse?
- e. Does community get along with adjacent communities? Do people collaborate on any community projects?

   f.  Do neighbors seem to support each other?
   g.  Community get-togethers?

Examination
   a.  Observation of interactions (generally or at specific meetings).
   b.  Statistics on interpersonal violence.
   c.  Statistics on employment, income, poverty.
   d.  Divorce rate.

## 9. SEXUALITY–REPRODUCTIVE PATTERN

History (Community Representatives)
   a.  Average family size?
   b.  Do people feel there are any problems with pornography, prostitution, other?
   c.  Do people want/support sex education in schools/community?

Examination
   a.  Family sizes and types of households.
   b.  Male/female ratio.
   c.  Average maternal age, maternal mortality rate, infant mortality rate.
   d.  Teen pregnancy rate.
   e.  Abortion rate.
   f.  Sexual violence statistics.
   g.  Laws/regulations regarding information on birth control.

## 10. COPING–STRESS-TOLERANCE PATTERN

History (Community Representatives)
   a.  Any groups that seem to be under stress?
   b.  Need/availability of phone help lines? Support groups (health related, other)?

Examination
   a.  Statistics on delinquency, drug abuse, alcoholism, suicide, psychiatric illness.
   b.  Unemployment rate by race, ethnic group, gender.

## 11. VALUE–BELIEF PATTERN

History (Community Representatives)

a. Community values: What seem to be the top four things that people living here see as important in their lives (note health-related values, priorities)?

b. Do people tend to get involved in causes/local fund-raising campaigns (note whether any are health related)?

c. Are there religious groups in the community? Churches available?

d. Do people tend to tolerate or not tolerate differences or socially deviant behavior?

Examination

a. Zoning/conservation laws.

b. Scan of community government health committee reports (goals, priorities).

c. Health budget relative to total budget.

## CRITICAL CARE ASSESSMENT

Clients who are critically ill, such as those with severe respiratory, cardiac, neurological, or psychological instability, are unable to respond to a full functional health pattern assessment. At times, examination and observation are the major data collection methods used during the critical phase of an illness. The client may not have the energy, capacity, or attention span to provide a health history. Nurses caring for critically ill individuals need to use screening techniques and be sensitive to cues of high-incidence diagnoses. Assessment of particular organ systems and other observational data would be added to the following items that screen for high-frequency/high-treatment-priority nursing diagnoses.

## FUNCTIONAL HEALTH PATTERNS ASSESSMENT GUIDELINES

### 1. HEALTH-PERCEPTION–HEALTH-MANAGEMENT PATTERN

   a. Risk for infection (break in skin from trauma or surgical incision, immunosuppression, debilitation, chronic disease, stasis of body fluids)? Specify area of risk (e.g., general or skin, respiratory, urinary).
   b. Risk for injury (impaired judgment, reduced level of consciousness, sensory-motor impairment, hearing and visual acuity, syncope, ability to use call light)?
   c. Understanding of health status (explanations needed)?

### 2. NUTRITIONAL–METABOLIC PATTERN

   a. Risk for nutritional deficit (intake/parenteral fluids, protein, vitamins, minerals)?
   b. Risk for pressure ulcer (bed mobility, skin over bony prominences, presence of restraints or casts, shear, friction, presence of traction)?
   c. Risk for ineffective thermoregulation (prematurity, head injury, hypothermia, hyperthermia)?
   d. Risk for fluid volume deficit (hypermetabolic states, intake-output)?
   e. Risk for aspiration (depressed cough and gag reflexes, level of consciousness, swallowing, gastric residual, tracheostomy, endotracheal tube)?

### 3. ELIMINATION PATTERN

   a. Risk for constipation/impaction (last bowel movement)?
   b. Risk for diarrhea, bowel incontinence?
   c. Urinary incontinence (catheter)?

### 4. ACTIVITY–EXERCISE PATTERN

   a. Risk for activity intolerance (respiratory, cardiac, circulatory problems; shortness of breath; dyspnea at rest or in-bed activities)?

  b.  Risk for ineffective airway clearance (on frequent suctioning; rhonchi, wheezes, moist rales, crackles; decreased breath sounds; respiratory problems)?
  c.  Ineffective breathing pattern (blood gases, respiratory rate and depth, compensatory position changes)?
  d.  Risk for joint contractures (immobilization—bed rest prolonged more than 24 hours, impaired bed mobility)?
  e.  Self-care deficit (level 1–4, total, or specify: bathing-hygiene, toileting, feeding, dressing-grooming)?
  f.  Risk for disuse syndrome (immobilization, paralysis, level of consciousness, 24-hour bed rest)?

## 5. SLEEP–REST PATTERN

  a.  Risk for sleep-pattern disturbance (concerns, fears, noise, interruptions, sleep-onset delay)?

## 6. COGNITIVE–PERCEPTUAL PATTERN

  a.  Sensory deficits (hearing, vision)?
  b.  Client/family decisional conflict (need for decisions, client's decision-making competency, treatment preferences documented)?
  c.  Impaired thought processes (confusion: general or nocturnal; hallucinations)?
  d.  Sensory deprivation or overload (monitors, isolation)?
  e.  Pain (report of severe discomfort/pain, guarding behavior, muscle tension, heart rate increases)?
  f.  Knowledge sufficient to reduce fear/anxiety (understanding of situation, treatments, care)?

## 7. SELF-PERCEPTION–SELF-CONCEPT PATTERN

  a.  Fear/anxiety (client verbal report, focus, family or other verbal report, focus of fear)?
  b.  Powerlessness (reported feelings of control or lack of control)?

    c. Hope (expresses hope or hopelessness)?

    d. Self-esteem/worth disturbance (expressions of guilt, perception of ability to deal with crisis)?

## 8. ROLE–RELATIONSHIP PATTERN

    a. Communication (verbal/nonverbal system, language)?

    b. Family processes/coping (when appropriate) (interactions, role adjustment, need for information, understanding of family role in the intensive care unit)?

    c. Grieving (when appropriate: perception of loss)?

    d. Role performance (emergency situations, e.g., child care responsibilities)?

    e. Parental role conflict (parental role confusion, family role conflicts)?

## 9. SEXUALITY–REPRODUCTIVE PATTERN

    a. Usually deferred unless pertains to the client's condition.

## 10. COPING–STRESS-TOLERANCE PATTERN

    a. Coping (anxiety level of client, family; compromised, disabling)?

## 11. VALUE–BELIEF PATTERN

    a. Spiritual distress (questions meanings, e.g., of suffering; inner conflict about beliefs; anger, nightmares, sleep disturbance)?

# Use of Diagnostic Categories in Clinical Practice

# USE OF DIAGNOSTIC CATEGORIES IN CLINICAL PRACTICE

Nursing diagnoses, in conjunction with medical diagnoses, provide a focus for most nursing care activities. Because issues of cost containment, case management, reimbursement, and quality assessment and improvement play such a large part in professional practice models, the following clinical applications of the diagnostic categories contained in this manual are suggested.

## DIAGNOSIS AND TREATMENT WITHIN THE NURSING PROCESS

a. The nursing process is a problem-identification and problem-solving process. The process is initiated with assessment (as the information collected provides cues to the health of an individual, family, or community).

Some cues are diagnostic. *A diagnostic cue is a critical defining characteristic, or clinical indicator, of a functional, dysfunctional, or potentially dysfunctional health state.* Consider a diagnostic cue important until investigation of its meaning proves otherwise. Use diagnostic categories as possible explanations of the meaning of cues. Consider alternative possible meanings for a cue or cue cluster (e.g., anxiety, fear, and depression).

b. Investigate the most likely possibilities first. Assess the presence or absence of diagnostic cues. These cues are the criteria that must be present before the diagnostic label is used; they are few in number.

c. Investigate the probable causes of the problem. Determine the etiological and/or related factors that, if altered, would have the greatest positive effect. Focus intervention on these factors first (e.g., self-care deficit, level III, related to activity intolerance). Avoid premature closure; be sure diagnostic cues are present to justify the diagnostic statement (problem and etiology).

d.  Determine the outcome/goal. The outcome represents the resolution of the problem or progress toward resolution. Specify time to resolution/evaluation. The time to resolution is influenced by the etiological/related factors.

e.  Syndromes do not have etiological or related factors specified. The probable cause is built into the diagnostic label (e.g., see posttraumatic, rape, translocation, disuse, sudden infant death).

f.  Risk diagnoses have risk factors. Intervene on the risk factors that can have the greatest impact in preventing the condition. Focus intervention on these factors first. Risk diagnoses do not have etiological/related factors.

g.  Wellness diagnoses with the title (Readiness for Enhanced, etc.) do not have etiological factors. They represent a client's desire to move to higher levels of wellness.

The key role of nursing diagnosis in nursing process may be seen in the diagram on pp. 40–41; it depicts the components of the nursing process.

## DOCUMENTATION

Use diagnostic category labels to describe the problem or potential problem. Use the client reports and observations to describe subjective and objective data (if a problem-oriented format is used). Etiological or related factors document the probable cause(s) that focuses nursing care planning. (Conditions currently not on accepted diagnostic listings should be documented in descriptive terms and subjected to clinical study.) Diagnoses, diagnosis-specific interventions, and diagnosis-specific outcomes are sufficiently developed for incorporating into computerized systems.

# USE OF DIAGNOSTIC CATEGORIES IN CLINICAL PRACTICE

## COMMUNICATION

Use diagnostic category labels as a concise summary of the client's condition in shift and administrative reports, discharge planning, referrals, and case conferences.

## CONSULTATIONS

Use cues and/or diagnostic category labels as a concise summary when requesting clinical nurse–specialist consultation. Diagnostic category labels are also useful when requesting consultation and specialized services to treat nursing diagnoses (e.g., nutritional, physical, occupational, recreational, art/music therapy). The consultant's report is also written using nursing diagnostic terms.

## QUALITY, STANDARDS OF CARE, AND NATIONAL GUIDELINES

Use diagnostic categories and their components as topics for process and outcome audits in a quality-improvement program. Assess the use of diagnoses and the accuracy of diagnostic judgments (process audit). Establish treatment guidelines for diagnoses, that is, intervention and outcome standards and criteria for their measurement. Implement national guidelines focusing on nursing diagnoses (pain, decubitus ulcer, depression, etc.) and developed by the United States Agency for Healthcare Research and Quality (see their website).

## COST OF NURSING CARE, REIMBURSEMENT, AND STAFFING

Diagnostic categories can be used as the focus of client classification. This is necessary for costing out nursing care, reimbursement, and staffing decisions. In determining cost of services, it is necessary to obtain a refined measure of resources consumed, such as that provided by nursing diagnoses. Determining cost of treatment based on nursing diagnosis, medical diagnosis, and an acuity factor is currently in the experimental stage.

## CASE MANAGEMENT

Diagnostic category labels are used in conjunction with medical diagnoses to focus case management. Nursing diagnosis–specific outcomes and medical diagnosis–specific outcomes are used in outcome-focused case management.

## CRITICAL PATHS

Nursing diagnostic categories and client strengths (identified during functional assessment) (1) describe variances that influence the path to a projected outcome for a disease or (2) are the basis for the construction of a nursing diagnosis critical path (with other nursing and medical diagnoses as variances). Critical paths are a way of scheduling recovery (attainment of outcomes) within a time and process (intervention/evaluation) framework.

## RESEARCH AND THEORY DEVELOPMENT

Diagnostic categories and their components provide concise summaries of the underlying concepts. They are the focus of clinical nursing research and are used in midrange theory building within nursing science. Research on the effectiveness of interventions for nursing diagnoses is ongoing.

# COMPONENTS OF NURSING PROCESS

Select a conceptual framework model of the client

Human functional health patterns

Assess patterns

EXIT or CONTINUE ASSESSMENT

NO

Signs and symptoms of dysfunctional patterns

Deviations from expected norms?

YES

Analyze and synthesize data; generate diagnostic hypothesis

Test diagnostic hypothesis

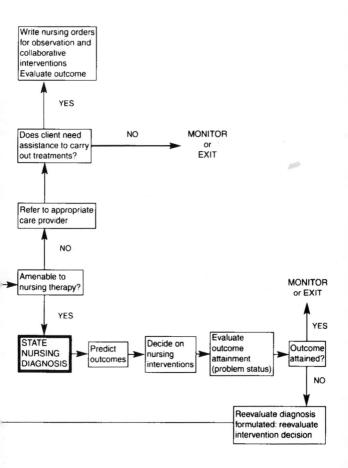

41

# Documentation:
# Format and Example

# DOCUMENTATION: FORMAT AND EXAMPLE

After an admission assessment, nursing diagnoses and treatment plans are documented in the client's record. Documentation is critically important for legal purposes, continuity of care, costing-out nursing services, reimbursement, and planning staffing of units. Currently, there is a transition from paper charts and a Kardex to computerized documentation in an electronic information system.

A commonly used documentation method, the problem-oriented record, is useful for both students and expert clinicians. This paper or electronic format for documentation provides (1) an indexing system for easy retrieval of information, (2) checkpoints for self-evaluation of diagnostic and therapeutic judgments, and (3) a master problem list (client problems listed by number) to increase coordination of treatment plans among care providers. As the example on pp. 52–55 illustrates, it includes the problem, supporting data, and the plan of care. Each diagnosis is given a number and entered on the master problem list. Following the documentation of the admission nursing history and examination, the problem number, nursing diagnosis, clinical data, and plan are recorded. Guidelines for recording are on pp. 45–47. The same problem number is used for all subsequent charting on a specific nursing diagnosis. An example of recording a nursing history and examination, diagnoses, and treatment plans using a paper-based method is on pp. 47–55.

Subjective or objective data related to a disease or its treatment are documented in the client's record by number (e.g., #2 Diabetes mellitus). Relabeling of the medical problem to document the related nursing care is not necessary (e.g., alteration in glucose metabolism or alteration in cardiac output). In fact, *relabeling in an indexing system leads to communication errors.*

In some clinical settings without computerized records, a Kardex is used; nursing diagnoses (problem/etiology), treatments, and outcomes are listed on the Kardex. Medical diagnoses, doctor's orders, and any related nursing orders with regard to observation or monitoring, drugs, treatments, and standard diagnostic and treatment protocols are also placed on the Kardex. Additional nursing orders, such as those related to observation of disease or individualization of disease treatments, are also listed on the Kardex. These nursing orders are within the collaborative domain of nursing practice and do not alter the medical treatment of disease.

With these methods of documentation, the client's record will reflect nursing judgments, actions, and evaluations relative to nursing and medical diagnoses. The Kardex will serve as a quick reference to all client problems that require nursing attention.

## PROBLEM-ORIENTED RECORDING GUIDELINES AND CHECKPOINTS

#___ PROBLEM NUMBER AND LABEL—State clear, concise diagnostic label for the problem.

Check below that S and O contain sufficient clinical data (diagnostic characteristics) for the problem.

If insufficient information is available, record the possible diagnoses being considered or the major signs/symptoms; continue assessment.

S: SUBJECTIVE DATA—List pertinent diagnostic indicators from verbal reports of individual or family.

Record quotes when applicable.

Check for consistency with objective data. Attempt to resolve incongruities or inconsistencies in data before recording.

O: OBJECTIVE DATA—List pertinent diagnostic indicators from direct observation and examination of individual or family, observations of context or milieu, and observational reports of other care providers, if pertinent.

Check for measurement error, observer bias, and consistency with subjective data. Attempt to resolve

incongruities or inconsistencies in data before
recording.

Note: S and O data must provide sufficient diagnostic
criteria to support problem and etiological factors.
See individual diagnosis pages to check defining
characteristics.

A: ASSESSMENT—State etiological or related factors
contributing to the problem in # _____.

Use clear, concise terms.

Check that S and O data provide diagnostic characteristics for etiological factor(s). If information available is insufficient to label etiological factors,
record possible factors being considered; continue
assessment.

May include functional strengths pertinent to resolution of the problem and any relevant prognostic
statements.

High-risk diagnoses do not have etiological factors;
the risk factors recorded in S and O are the factors
contributing to the high-risk state. They are the focus for the plan of care.

P: PLAN—State projected outcome(s) and interventions.

Projected outcome(s): state concise, explicit, measurable,
critical, attainable outcome(s) for the problem. State time
of outcome attainment (e.g., discharge, 3 days, 4-week
visit). If applicable, state a sequential set of outcomes
and time frame.

Check that outcomes are specific to problem in
# _____.

Check that date of outcome attainment is realistic.
Consider etiological factors that may influence
time for outcome attainment.

Interventions: State intervention goal (optional). List
concise nursing treatment orders. Include specific
actions (time and amount, if applicable).

Check that treatment orders are consistent with cause
stated in A and are specific to the individual client.
If there is a potential problem with no etiological
factor, check that treatment orders will reduce risk
factors specified under S and O.

Check that treatment orders have a high possibility
for attaining outcome(s).

If useful, classify plan by treatment orders (P-rx), diagnostic orders (P-dx), and teaching orders (P-ed).

## EXAMPLE: NURSING HISTORY AND EXAMINATION

The following is an example of documentation of a nursing
history and examination. Note that the first section has a
few introductory sentences that alerts the reader to the age,
gender, marital state, medical condition, and general appearance, race, and ethnic background when appropriate. Within
this framework is information that suggests what norms are
to be applied in judging whether a health pattern is functional, dysfunctional, or potentially dysfunctional.

## NURSING HISTORY

First hospital admission of a 55-year-old, married, obese, ad-
ministrator of a Spanish center. Sitting upright in bed, tense
posture and expression. Five-year history of slightly elevated
blood pressure. One-year PTA dizziness lasted 12 hours and
started on medication; two other episodes relieved by rest.
Seeks treatment at emergency room for dizziness and numbness of left arm.

### Health-Perception–Health-Management Pattern

Viewed health as good until 1 year ago when diagnosed as
having "high blood pressure." States job is "stressful, but the
people need me." Had headaches for last 6 months and two
episodes of dizziness, one at work and one at home lasting
about 2 hours. Rested and symptoms went away. Delayed

seeking care because was "too busy." Thought it was "overwork," not blood pressure. Discontinued blood pressure
medication and visits to doctor about 6 months ago, "when
blood pressure came down and I felt better"; states medicine
caused impotence. Came to emergency room today because
of left arm numbness and fear of stroke. Mother died of
"stroke" 15 months ago. Concerned that he hasn't been taking care of himself and "I need to learn about what to do."
Wants to know "everything." Asked whether it is okay to do
some job-related paperwork if someone brought it in. Takes
no medicine currently, except Alka-Seltzer and a laxative;
doesn't smoke; drinks socially.

### Nutritional–Metabolic Pattern

Sample diet related: MDR (minimum daily requirement) intake of protein, excess carbohydrate and fat; minimal high-
roughage foods (fruits and vegetables), approximately 3 cups
of coffee/day, fluid intake low, no history of lesions at mouth
corners or mucous membranes; has gained weight gradually
last 15 years. Some indigestion and heartburn after lunch attributed to days with multiple problems; takes Alka-Seltzer;
dieting unsuccessful; problem is, "probably stress of job; I get
home and eat a big supper and snacks in the evening"; no
food dislikes. Takes lunch (sandwich and cake) to work and
eats at desk; restaurants in area not good.

### Elimination Pattern

Daily bowel movement pattern with two or three episodes of
constipation/month lasting 2 days, hard stools, straining,
and laxatives used. Attributes this pattern to his diet; knows
he should eat better. Reports no problems voiding or in control of elimination.

### Activity–Exercise Pattern

Spectator sports, uses car, minimal walking because of time
schedule, sedentary job, considers self too old for exercise.

Increasing fatigue last few weeks, less energy 2 months before admission; no self care deficit. Recreation consists of reading novels, watching television, dinner with other couples. Lives in first-floor apartment in city, and drives 3/4 mile to work.

### Sleep–Rest Pattern

Average 4 to 6 hours sleep/night, quiet atmosphere, own room with wife, double bed, uses bed board. Presleep activities include watching television or completing paperwork from job; difficulty with sleep onset 1 month; awakens in morning many times thinking about job-related problems.

### Cognitive–Perceptual Pattern

Sight corrected with glasses, changed 1 year ago; no change in hearing, taste, smell. No perceived change in memory, "I couldn't take it if I started losing my mind, like with a stroke." Learning ability: sees self as slower than in college, alert manner, grasps questions easily. Takes no sedatives, tranquilizers, other drugs. No headache at present.

### Self-Perception–Self-Concept Pattern

Sees self as needing to do things well (job, father, husband). "Sometimes don't think I'm doing well with my family—having them live in this area—but in my job you have to be near when people need help." "It will be just great if I get sick and they have to take care of me, instead of me taking care of them."

### Role–Relationship Pattern

Describes family as happy and understanding of his job commitments, wife formerly a social worker; kids "good, but I know we'll have trouble as Joe (10 years old) gets older." "Maybe I should move us out of [lower socioeconomic area in city cited]." Ten-year-old assaulted 4 months ago; 14-year-old boy interested in sports and "keeps out of trouble, so far." Family usually "sits down together" to handle problems. Social

relationships confined to "a few other couples"; finds this sufficient. Job demanding 9–10 hours/day, "always trying to get
money to keep the center solvent" (assistant taking over while
in hospital). Enjoys job and helping people; coworkers are
"good to work with." Wife states that they are close; worried
about husband's health; states he is more concerned with
other people than himself. She admires him for this. Wife able
to handle home responsibilities during hospitalization. States
she and children had physical examination recently; no health
problems; no elevation in blood pressure.

### Sexuality–Reproductive Pattern

Two children; states was impotent when on BP medication.
When "BP went down" stopped medications; potency
returned. No problems perceived in sexual relationship.

### Coping–Stress-Tolerance Pattern

Feels tense at work; has tried relaxation exercises with some
alleviation; doesn't always have time. States the best way to
deal with problems is to "attack them." Afraid of having a
stroke and being dependent. "This thing today has really
scared me." "I have too many things to think about at work
and at home, and now this blood pressure thing." Life
changes: father died 3 years ago; mother died of stroke
15 months ago. Took job at Spanish center 2 years ago to
be near mother who "was getting old." Pleased he did this
and feels good about it.

### Value–Belief Pattern

"Life has been good to me"; feels deeply about "injustices in
society" and wants to do something about them. States family is important to him. Religion (Catholic) important to
him; would like to be active in church affairs.

## DOCUMENTATION: FORMAT AND EXAMPLE

### EXAMINATION

Blood pressure ___205/118___ Temperature ___99.8___
Pulse rate __Regular and strong__ Respirations ___18___

### NUTRITIONAL–METABOLIC PATTERN

Skin _____No redness over bony prominence; no lesions_____
Oral mucous membranes _____Moist; no lesions_____
Actual weight __230__ Reported weight __220__ Height __5'11"__

### ACTIVITY-EXERCISE PATTERN

Gait _____Steady_____ Posture _____Well balanced_____
Muscle tone, strength-coordination __Left and right hand grip firm;__
lifts both legs; can pick up pencil; tension in neck and shoulder
muscles
Range-of-motion (joints) Some tightness when bending forward
Prostheses/assistive devices _____None_____
Absence of body part _____No_____
Demonstrated ability for:
Feeding _____0_____ Grooming _____0_____
Bathing _____0_____ General mobility _____0_____
Toileting _____0_____ Dressing _____0_____
(0 = full self care)

### COGNITIVE-PERCEPTUAL PATTERN

Perceptual: Hears whisper _Yes_ Reads newsprint _With glasses_
Language ___English; grasps concrete and abstract ideas, Speech__
clear. Attention span good.

### SELF-PERCEPTION–SELF-CONCEPT PATTERN

General appearance _____Well groomed; good hygiene_____
Nervous/relaxed __2 (scale of 1–5 with 1 = relaxed) Tension__
decreased during history taking
Eye contact _____Yes_____ Attention span _____Good_____
Assertive/passive _____3 (scale of 1–5 with 1 = passive)_____

# DOCUMENTATION: FORMAT AND EXAMPLE

## ROLE–RELATIONSHIP PATTERN

Interactions <u>Communications with wife supportive; both somewhat</u>
<u>tense; children not present</u>

## PROBLEM LIST

### 1  Exogenous Obesity

S: Reports diet of excess carbohydrate and fat; big supper, evening snack, sandwich and cake at lunch, eats
at desk. Reports gradual weight gain last 15 years;
considers self too old for exercise; sedentary job;
spectator sports, drives 3/4 mile to work. Reports
220 lbs.

O: 59110, 230 lbs. Dryness, calluses on feet with
discomfort when walking. Current diet order:
1,200 calories.

A: Caloric intake–energy expenditure imbalance. Reports
dieting unsuccessful in past; discomfort when walking
may reduce exercise.

Discharge outcome: (1) Writes 1-week's 1200-calorie diet
using calorie guide, (2) states how meal plan can be
carried out within daily routine, and (3) states plan
for increasing exercise and amount of weight loss to
be achieved per month.

P: Discuss why dieting previously unsuccessful. Assess
motivation, readiness, and current plans for weight
loss; develop educational plan to achieve outcomes.
Suggest podiatrist.

### 2  Intermittent Constipation Pattern

S: Daily bowel movement with two or three episodes
of constipation per month; constipation lasts 2 days,
hard stools, straining, laxatives used; attributes this
to minimal high-roughage foods, low fluid intake;
minimal walking, exercise; no constipation reported
at present.

A: Dietary-Exercise Pattern

Discharge outcome: (1) Daily bowel movement without straining, and (2) states a plan for increasing fluid intake and high-fiber foods in diet.

P: Check qd bowel pattern in hospital. Provide supplementary fluids between meals. Integrate teaching of fluid and high-fiber food requirements into weight loss dietary teaching (see Problem 1).

### 3  Fear (Dependency)

S: "Couldn't take it if started losing my mind, like with a stroke." "Just great if I get sick and they have to take care of me, instead of me taking care of them." States fear of stroke and becoming dependent—"this thing today has scared me"; mother died of stroke 15 months ago. States best way to deal with problems is to "attack them."

O: Neck and shoulder muscles tense.

A: Perceived risk of stroke.

Outcome, day 2: (1) neck and shoulder muscles relaxed, and (2) identifies ways to reduce future risk of dependency (stroke).

P: Orient to environment and explain procedures (cognitive and sensory orientation). Back massage for relaxation q4h for 2 days. Allow to verbalize fears of dependency and channel thinking toward "attacking" risk factors; integrate discussion with dietary planning and conflict resolution.

### 4  Value Conflict

S: Feels deeply about injustices in society; wants to do something about them; head of Spanish center in inner city; enjoys job and helping people; coworkers good; job demanding, 9–10 hours/day; always trying to get money to keep Spanish center solvent; "job

stressful, but people need me"; feels tense at work—
tried relaxation; doesn't always have time to relax;
4 to 6 hours sleep/night, sleep onset difficulty 1 month,
presleep activities include job-related paperwork; awakens thinking about job-related problems.

Wife states he's more concerned with others than
himself—admires him for this; kids "good, but know
we'll have trouble as Joe gets older"; "maybe I should
move"; 10-year-old assaulted 4 months ago; sees self
as needing to do things well (job, father, husband);
sometimes thinks "not doing well with my family—
having them live in this area—but in my job you have
to be near when people need help"; "I have too many
things to think about at work, and at home, and now
this blood pressure thing."

O: BP 205/118; 5-year history of essential hypertension.

A: Perceived responsibilities (job and family, possibly self)

Discharge outcome: States plan for periodically assessing
commitments/priorities in life.

P: Assess time constraints relative to valued activities
(job, family, health management responsibilities).
Help determine high-priority responsibilities (clarify
values). Discuss possibility that time allocation to valued areas may resolve conflicts. Discuss value of
health management so can continue to help others
and realize goals. Consider nursing referral.

### Risk Prone Health Behavior*

S: Delayed seeking care because "too busy"; attributed
headaches and dizziness to overwork; stopped medicines and follow-up care "when BP went down"; states
impotent on BP medicines.

---

*It may be possible to cluster all other problems under Risk Prone Health
Behavior related to Perceived Responsibilities and Priorities. The care objective
would be to help the client examine his values (priorities) and to balance job,
family, and health-management responsibilities.

O: BP 205/118; 59110, 230 lbs.

A: May be motivated to improve health management at this time; states he wants to learn what to do.

Discharge outcome: States how daily routine will be adapted to implement health management plans (medication regimen, diet-exercise, bowel, and value–conflict management).

P: Assess motivation and readiness to improve health management; develop plan for learning management of hypertension, diet, exercise, elimination, and value conflict (the general plan of hypertensive and transient ischemic attack management can be reviewed until specific drugs, etc., are prescribed for discharge).

## Hypertension with Evidence of Transient Ischemic Attack (Medical Diagnosis Made and Recorded by Physician)

P: Lisinopril 20 mg bid; 1,200-calorie diet with no added salt; BP q4h; medical orders: notify doctor if diastolic greater than 100, severe headache, dizziness. Observe for weakness in muscles of face or extremities and notify doctor (nursing order).

# Diagnostic
# Categories

# Health-Perception–
# Health-Management
# Pattern

## Risk-Prone Health Behavior  2006, 2008

**DEFINITION**

Failure to modify lifestyle/behaviors in a manner that improves health status

**DEFINING CHARACTERISTICS**

**Diagnostic Cues**

- Failure to take action that prevents health problems
- Minimizes health status change

and/or

- Demonstrates nonacceptance of health status change

**Supporting Cues**

- Failure to achieve optimal sense of control

**OUTCOME**

**Acceptance: Health Status**

- Adjusts lifestyle/behaviors to attain optimal health and well-being

**ETIOLOGICAL OR RELATED FACTORS**

- Inadequate comprehension
- Inadequate social support
- Low self-efficacy
- Low socioeconomic status
- Multiple stressors
- Negative attitude toward health care
- Excessive alcohol ingestion; smoking

**HIGH-RISK POPULATIONS**

- Multiple responsibilities
- History of perceived invulnerability

## Ineffective Health Maintenance (Specify)* (1982)

### DEFINITION

Inability to identify basic health practices, manage own health, or seek help to maintain health

### DEFINING CHARACTERISTICS

#### Diagnostic Cues

+ Demonstrated lack of knowledge regarding basic health practices (inability to state this knowledge) and/or
+ Reported or observed inability to take responsibility for meeting basic health practices in any or all functional pattern areas

#### Supporting Cues

+ History of lack of health-seeking behavior
+ Expression of interest in improving health behaviors
+ Demonstrated lack of adaptive behaviors to internal or external changes

### OUTCOME

#### Personal Health Status

+ Overall physical, psychological, social, and spiritual functioning meets expected norms

### ETIOLOGICAL OR RELATED FACTORS

+ Unachieved developmental tasks
+ Complete or partial lack of gross/fine motor skills

*Continues*

---

*Note: The definition specifies inability (physical or mental) to manage own health; use other diagnoses if this ability is present. See Noncompliance, Health Management Deficit, Risk Prone Health Behavior.

## Ineffective Health Maintenance (Specify) (1982)—cont'd

- Uncompensated perceptual–cognitive impairment (perception and judgment)
- Ineffective coping (individual or family)
- Disabling spiritual distress
- Dysfunctional grieving
- Reported or observed lack of material resources (equipment, finances, or other resources for health maintenance)
- Reported or observed impairment of personal support system

### HIGH-RISK POPULATIONS

- Mental retardation
- Cognitive impairment (e.g., severe head injury, Alzheimer's disease, dementia, and other mental disorders)
- Sensory-motor impairment (e.g., hemiplegia, paraplegia)

## Ineffective Health Management* (2008)

### DEFINITION

Pattern of regulating and integrating into daily living a therapeutic regime for treatment of illness and its sequelae that is unsatisfactory for meeting specific health goals

### DEFINING CHARACTERISTICS

- Failure to include treatment regimens in daily living
- Verbalizes difficulty with prescribed regimens
- Verbalizes desire to manage illness
- Failure to take action to reduce risk factors
- Choices in daily living are ineffective for meeting health goals

### OUTCOME

#### Health-Promoting Behavior

- Consistently demonstrates personal actions that promote wellness and/or manage therapeutic regimen to meet health goals
- States plan for integrating therapeutic regimen or rehabilitative recommendations into daily activities (prior to assuming responsibility for self management)

### ETIOLOGICAL OR RELATED FACTORS

- Complexity of healthcare system
- Complexity of therapeutic regimen
- Decisional conflicts
- Economic difficulties
- Excessive demands made (e.g., individual, family)
- Family conflict
- Family patterns of health care

*Continues*

*Note: Name changed from the NANDA-I (Self Health Management to Health Management).

### Ineffective Health Management (2008)—*cont'd*

- Inadequate number of cues to action
- Knowledge deficit
- Perceived barriers
- Powerlessness
- Perceived seriousness
- Perceived low susceptibility; lack of benefit
- Social support deficit
- New treatment regimen
- Mental retardation

## HIGH-RISK POPULATIONS

- New and/or complex treatment regime

## Readiness for Enhanced Health Management* (2008)

### DEFINITION

A pattern of regulating and integrating into daily living a therapeutic regime for treatment of illness and its sequelae that is sufficient for meeting health-related goals and can be strengthened

### DEFINING CHARACTERISTICS

- ♦ Choices of daily living are appropriate for meeting goals (e.g., treatment, prevention)
- ♦ Describes reduction of risk factors
- ♦ Expresses desire to manage the illness (e.g., treatment, prevention of sequelae)
- ♦ Expresses little difficulty with prescribed regimens
- ♦ No unexpected acceleration of illness symptoms

### OUTCOME

#### Health-Promoting Behavior

- ♦ Consistently demonstrates personal actions that promote wellness and/or manage therapeutic regimen to meet health goals
- ♦ States plan for integrating therapeutic regimen or rehabilitative recommendations into daily activities

*Note: Name changed from the NANDA-I (Self Health Management to Health Management).

## Ineffective Therapeutic Regimen Management (Specify Area)

### DEFINITION

Pattern of regulating/integrating into daily living a program for treatment of illness and its sequelae that is not meeting specific health goals (specify medication, activity, other treatment regimens, or health promotion/disease prevention)

### DEFINING CHARACTERISTICS

#### Diagnostic Cues

- Report or observation that specific health goals are not met (specify goals) and one of the following:
- States that did not take action to include treatment regimens in daily routines
- States did not take action to reduce risk factors for progression of illness and sequelae

#### Supporting Cues

- Choices about daily living ineffective for meeting goals of a treatment or prevention program (specify)
- Acceleration (expected or unexpected) of illness symptoms
- Verbalizes difficulty with regulation/integration of one or more prescribed regimens for treatment of illness or illness effects or for prevention of complications
- Expresses desire to manage the treatment of illness or prevention of sequelae

### OUTCOME

#### Compliance Behavior

- Takes personal actions to promote wellness, recovery, and rehabilitation based on professional advice

# HEALTH-PERCEPTION–HEALTH-MANAGEMENT PATTERN

## ETIOLOGICAL OR RELATED FACTORS

+ Complexity of therapeutic regimen
+ Low perceived seriousness
+ Perceived low susceptibility
+ Perceived barriers (specify)
+ Perceived cost exceeds benefits
+ Mistrust (specify; e.g., of regimen or healthcare personnel)
+ Decisional conflict (specify)
+ Economic difficulties
+ Excessive demands (individual/family)
+ Family conflict
+ Family patterns of health care (specify)
+ Inadequate cues to action (number/types)
+ Knowledge deficit (specify)
+ Social support deficits
+ Complexity of healthcare system

## HIGH-RISK POPULATIONS

+ New treatment regimen
+ Mental retardation
+ Alzheimer's disease, dementia, and other mental disorders
+ Sensory-motor impairment (e.g., hemiplegia, paraplegia)
+ Severe head injury

# HEALTH-PERCEPTION–HEALTH-MANAGEMENT PATTERN

### Risk for Ineffective Therapeutic Regimen Management (Specify Area)*

## DEFINITION

Presence of risk factors for difficulty in regulating/integrating a treatment or prevention program into daily living

## RISK FACTORS

- Perceived low susceptibility/seriousness
- Perceived barriers (specify; e.g., value, cultural, or spiritual conflict)
- Perceived cost exceeds benefits
- Mistrust (specify; e.g., of regimen/healthcare personnel)
- Powerlessness
- Complexity of therapeutic regimen
- Decisional conflict (specify)
- Economic difficulties
- Excessive demands made on individual/family
- Family conflict
- Family patterns of health care (specify)
- Inadequate cues to action (number/types)
- Knowledge deficit (specify)
- Social support deficit
- Complexity of healthcare system
- Severe depression
- Impaired reality testing
- Uncompensated visual or hearing loss
- Uncompensated memory deficit
- Impaired mobility/coordination
- Activity intolerance
- Value conflict/priority setting
- Denial of illness

*See also Noncompliance, Ineffective Health Management, Ineffective Health Maintenance.

68

## OUTCOME

### Compliance Behavior

♦ Takes personal actions to promote wellness, recovery, and rehabilitation based on professional advice

## Ineffective Family Therapeutic Regimen Management (Specify Area) (1994)

### DEFINITION

Pattern of regulating and integrating into family processes a program for treatment of illness and the sequelae of illness that is unsatisfactory for meeting specific health goals

### DEFINING CHARACTERISTICS

+ Inappropriate family activities for meeting the goals of a treatment or prevention program
+ Acceleration of illness symptoms of a family member
+ Lack of attention to illness and its sequelae
+ Verbalized desire to manage the treatment of illness and prevention of the sequelae
+ Verbalized difficulty with regulation/integration of one or more effects or prevention of complication
+ Verbalizes that family did not take action to reduce risk factors for progression of illness and sequelae

### OUTCOME

#### Family Normalization

+ Capacity of the family to maintain routines and develop strategies for optimal functioning when a member has a chronic illness or disability

### ETIOLOGICAL OR RELATED FACTORS

+ Complexity of healthcare system
+ Complexity of therapeutic regimen
+ Decisional conflicts
+ Economic difficulties
+ Excessive demands made on individual or family
+ Family conflict

## Ineffective Community Therapeutic Regimen Management (Specify Area) (1994)

### DEFINITION

Pattern of regulating and integrating into community processes programs for treatment of illness and sequelae of illness that are unsatisfactory for meeting health-related goals

### DEFINING CHARACTERISTICS

- ♦ Deficits in accountability of persons and programs for illness care of aggregates (primary, secondary, and tertiary prevention)
- ♦ Deficits in advocates for aggregates
- ♦ Illness symptoms above the norm expected for the number and type of population
- ♦ Number of healthcare resources are insufficient or unavailable for the prevalence of illness(s)
- ♦ Unexpected acceleration of illness(s)

### OUTCOME

### Community Risk Control (Type)

- ♦ Community actions taken to prevent, eliminate, or reduce modifiable health threats

## Health Management Deficit (Specify Area)

### DEFINITION

Inability to manage activities related to health promotion and/or disease or disability prevention/progression (specify drug or treatment regimen, dietary prescription, observation and reporting of symptoms, follow-up care of disease, health promotion, and disease prevention)

### DEFINING CHARACTERISTICS

#### Diagnostic Cues

One or more of the following:

- Report or observation of inability to manage treatment regimen
- Report or observation of inability to manage mental or physical health–promotion activities specific to age and developmental stage
- Report or observation of insufficient actions to prevent diseases or disabilities that pose a risk to the individual or family

### OUTCOME

#### Compliance Behavior

- Takes personal actions to promote wellness, recovery, and rehabilitation based on professional advice

### ETIOLOGICAL OR RELATED FACTORS

- Knowledge deficit (specify area)
- Priority setting (values)
- Parental care priorities
- Severe depression
- Impaired reality testing
- Uncompensated memory deficit
- Impaired mobility (levels II through IV)

- Uncompensated impaired coordination
- Uncompensated perceptual or cognitive impairment
- Activity intolerance (levels III or IV)

## HIGH-RISK POPULATIONS

- New and/or complex treatment regimen
- Mental retardation
- Cognitive impairment (e.g., severe head injury, Alzheimer's disease, dementia, and other mental disorders)
- Sensory-motor impairment (e.g., hemiplegia, paraplegia)

## Risk for Health-Management Deficit (Specify Area)

### DEFINITION

Presence of risk factors for inability to manage activities related to health promotion and/or disease or disability prevention (specify drug or treatment regimen, dietary prescription, observation and reporting of symptoms, follow-up care of disease, health promotion, disease prevention)

### RISK FACTORS

+ Priority setting, knowledge, comprehension, and/or motor skills needed for continuing treatment of disease exceed actual or potential competencies
+ Priority setting, knowledge, comprehension, and/or motor skills required for specific health promotion and disease prevention activities exceed actual or potential competencies
+ Activity intolerance (level IV)
+ Uncompensated perceptual or cognitive impairment
+ Uncompensated impaired coordination
+ Impaired mobility (levels II through IV)
+ Uncompensated short-term memory deficit
+ Uncompensated visual or hearing loss
+ Impaired reality testing
+ Severe depression

### OUTCOME

#### Compliance Behavior

+ Takes personal actions to promote wellness, recovery, and rehabilitation based on professional advice

## Noncompliance (Specify Area) (1973, 1996, 1998)

### DEFINITION

Nonadherence to a therapeutic recommendation after informed decision and expressed intention to attain therapeutic goals (specify drug or treatment regimen, dietary prescription, observation and reporting of symptoms, follow-up care, health-promoting behaviors)

### DEFINING CHARACTERISTICS

#### Diagnostic Cues

One or more of the following:

- ◆ Direct observation of noncompliance or statements by client or significant others describing behaviors indicating failure to adhere
- ◆ Objective tests revealing nonadherence (physiological measures, detection of markers)

#### Supporting Cues

- ◆ Evidence of development of complications
- ◆ Evidence of exacerbation of symptoms
- ◆ Failure to keep appointments
- ◆ Failure to progress (resolve problem)

### OUTCOME

#### Adherence Behavior

- ◆ Takes self-initiated actions to promote wellness, recovery and rehabilitation

### ETIOLOGICAL OR RELATED FACTORS

- ◆ Value, health beliefs, cultural, or spiritual conflict
- ◆ Knowledge or skill deficit (developmental abilities)
- ◆ Perceived therapeutic ineffectiveness

*Continues*

**Noncompliance (Specify Area) (1973, 1996, 1998)—*cont'd***

+ Perceived nonsusceptibility or invulnerability
+ Denial of illness
+ Family pattern disruption
+ Low motivation
+ Satisfaction with care/credibility and continuity of provider/access and convenience of care/client–provider relationship

## HIGH-RISK POPULATIONS

+ New and/or complex treatment regimen (duration, cost, or complexity)

## Risk for Noncompliance (Specify Area)

### DEFINITION

Presence of risk factors for nonadherence to the therapeutic recommendations following informed decision and expressed intention to adhere or to attain therapeutic goals

### RISK FACTORS

- Denial of illness
- Perceived ineffectiveness of recommended practices
- Perceived lack of seriousness of problem or risk factors
- Perceived lack of susceptibility
- Insufficient knowledge or skills (therapeutic recommendations)
- Absence of a plan for integrating therapeutic recommendations into daily routines
- New and/or complex treatment regimen
- Lack of support systems (supportive others)
- History of noncompliance with aspects of therapeutic regimen

### OUTCOME

#### Compliance Behavior

- Demonstrates personal actions to promote wellness, recovery, and/or rehabilitation based on professional advice

## Contamination (2007)

### DEFINITION

Exposure to environmental contaminants in doses sufficient to cause adverse health effects.

### DEFINING CHARACTERISTICS

(Defining characteristics are dependent on the causative agent. Agents cause a variety of individual organ responses as well as systemic responses.)

#### Pesticides

+ Dermatological effects of pesticide exposure
+ Gastrointestinal effects of pesticide exposure
+ Neurological effects of pesticide exposure
+ Pulmonary effects of pesticide exposure
+ Renal effects of pesticide exposure

(Major categories of pesticides: insecticides, herbicides, fungicides, antimicrobials, rodenticides; major pesticides: organophosphates, carbamates, organochlorines, pyrethrium, arsenic, glycophosphates, bipyridyls, chlorophenoxy)

#### Chemicals

+ Dermatological effects of chemical exposure
+ Gastrointestinal effects of chemical exposure
+ Immunologic effects of chemical exposure
+ Neurological effects of chemical exposure
+ Pulmonary effects of chemical exposure
+ Renal effects of chemical exposure

(Major categories of chemical agents: petroleum-based agents, anticholinesterases; type I agents act on proximal tracheobronchial portion of the respiratory tract; type II agents act on alveoli; type III agents produce systemic effects)

## HEALTH-PERCEPTION–HEALTH-MANAGEMENT PATTERN

### Biologics

- Dermatological effects of exposure to biologics
- Gastrointestinal effects of exposure to biologics
- Pulmonary effects of exposure to biologics
- Neurological effects of exposure to biologics
- Renal effects of exposure to biologics (toxins from living organisms ([bacteria, viruses, fungi])

### Pollution

- Neurological effects of pollution exposure
- Pulmonary effects of pollution exposure
- Major locations: air, water, soil; major agents: asbestos, radon, tobacco, heavy metal, lea, noise, exhaust

### Waste

- Dermatological effects of waste exposure
- Gastrointestinal effects of waste exposure
- Hepatic effects of waste exposure
- Pulmonary effects of waste exposure
- Categories of waste: trash, raw sewage, industrial waste

### Radiation

- Immunological effects of radiation exposure
- Genetic effects of radiation exposure
- Neurological effects of radiation exposure
- Oncologic effects of radiation exposure
- Categories: internal—exposure through ingestion of radioactive material (e.g., food/water contaminations); external—exposure through direct contact with radioactive material

*Continues*

**Contamination** (2007)—*cont'd*

## OUTCOME

* Resolution of systemic response to contamination (specify type)

## RELATED FACTORS

### External

* Chemical contamination of food
* Chemical contamination of water
* Exposure to bioterrorism
* Exposure to disaster (natural or man-made)
* Exposure to radiation (occupation in radiography, employment in nuclear industries and electrical generating plants, living near nuclear industries and electrical generating plants)
* Flaking, peeling paint in presence of young children
* Flaking, peeling plaster in presence of young children
* Flooring surface (carpeted surfaces hold contaminated residue more than hard floor surfaces)
* Geographic area (living in area where high level of contaminants exists)
* Household hygiene practices
* Inadequate municipal services (trash removal, sewage treatment facilities)
* Inappropriate use of protective clothing
* Lack of breakdown of contaminants once indoors (breakdown is inhibited without sun and rain exposure)
* Living in poverty (increases potential for multiple exposures, lack of access to health care, and poor diet)
* Paint, lacquer, etc. in poorly ventilated areas
* Paint, lacquer, etc. without effective protection
* Personal hygiene practices

- Playing in outdoor areas where environmental contaminants are used
- Presence of atmospheric pollutants
- Use of environmental contaminants in the home (e.g., pesticides, chemicals, environmental tobacco smoke)
- Unprotected contact with heavy metals or chemicals (e.g., arsenic, chromium, lead)

## Internal

- Age (children less than 5 years, older adults)
- Concomitant exposures
- Developmental characteristics of children
- Female gender
- Gestational age during exposure
- Nutritional factors (e.g., obesity, vitamin and mineral deficiencies)
- Pre-existing disease states
- Pregnancy
- Previous exposure
- Smoking

## Risk for Contamination (2007)

### DEFINITION

Accentuated risk for exposure to environmental contaminants in doses sufficient to cause adverse health effects

### RISK FACTORS

### External

- Chemical contamination of food
- Chemical contamination of water
- Exposure to bioterrorism
- Exposure to disaster (natural or man-made)
- Exposure to radiation (occupation in radiography, employment in nuclear industries and electrical generating plants, living near nuclear industries and electrical generating plants)
- Flaking, peeling paint in presence of young children
- Flaking, peeling plaster in presence of young children
- Flooring surface (carpeted surfaces hold contaminated residue more than hard floor surfaces)
- Geographic area (living in area where high level of contaminants exists)
- Household hygiene practices
- Inadequate municipal services (trash removal, sewage treatment facilities)
- Inappropriate use of protective clothing
- Lack of breakdown of contaminants once indoors (breakdown is inhibited without sun and rain exposure)
- Living in poverty (increases potential for multiple exposures, lack of access to health care, and poor diet)
- Paint, lacquer, and so forth in poorly ventilated areas
- Paint, lacquer, and so forth without effective protection
- Personal hygiene practices

- Playing in outdoor areas where environmental contaminants are used
- Presence of atmospheric pollutants
- Use of environmental contaminants in the home (e.g., pesticides, chemicals, environmental tobacco smoke)
- Unprotected contact with heavy metals or chemicals (e.g., arsenic, chromium, lead)

### Internal

- Age (children less than 5 years, older adults)
- Concomitant exposures
- Developmental characteristics of children
- Female gender
- Gestational age during exposure
- Nutritional factors (e.g., obesity, vitamin and mineral deficiencies)
- Pre-existing disease states
- Pregnancy
- Previous exposure
- Smoking

### OUTCOME

Absence of sources of contamination

## Readiness for Enhanced Immunization Status (2007)

### DEFINITION

Pattern of conforming to local, national, and/or international standards of immunization to prevent infectious disease(s) that is sufficient to protect a person, family, or community and can be strengthened

### DEFINING CHARACTERISTICS

- Expresses desire to enhance behavior to prevent infectious disease
- Expresses desire to enhance identification of possible problems associated with immunization
- Expresses desire to enhance identification of providers of immunization
- Expresses desire to enhance immunization status
- Expresses desire to enhance knowledge of immunization standards
- Expresses desire to enhance record-keeping of immunizations

### OUTCOME

**Personal Health Status**

- Overall physical, psychological, social, and spiritual functioning meets expected norms

## Risk for Infection (Specify Type/Area) (1986)

### DEFINITION

Presence of increased risk for invasion by pathogenic organisms (specify respiratory, urinary tract, skin)

### RISK FACTORS

- Tissue destruction (surgical wound, traumatized tissues, invasive procedure, bites, burns)
- Skin breakdown (e.g., pressure ulceration)
- Stasis of body fluids or secretions (e.g., bladder, lungs, sinuses)
- Immunosuppression (e.g., chemotherapy, steroids, stress, disease)
- Inadequate acquired immunity
- Increased environmental exposure to pathogens (specify type)
- Inadequate secondary defenses: leukopenia (e.g., radiation, chemotherapy)
- Decreased hemoglobin and oxygen transport, suppressed inflammatory response
- Chronic disease with debilitation
- Malnutrition; hyperglycemia
- Change in normal flora (antibiotic, antiviral, antifungal medicines)
- Decrease in ciliary action
- Insufficient knowledge to avoid exposure to pathogens
- Warm, moist, dark areas (e.g., skin folds)
- Rupture of amniotic membranes
- Altered peristalsis
- Change in pH of secretions

*Continues*

## Risk for Infection (Specify Type/Area) (1986)—*cont'd*

**Presence of stressors**

 ♦ Radiation therapy

**OUTCOME**

**Infection Severity**

 ♦ Absence of infection and associated symptoms

## Risk for Injury  (1978)

**DEFINITION**

Presence of risk factors for trauma to the body

**RISK FACTORS**

**Cognitive Factors**

- Excess alcohol-ingestion pattern
- Impaired judgment (disease, drugs, impaired reality testing, risk-taking behavior)
- Sensory-perceptual loss or deterioration (temperature, touch, position-sense, vision, hearing)
- Disorientation
- Unfamiliar setting
- Inability to use call light; inappropriate call-for-aid mechanisms

**Mobility Factors**

- Impaired mobility (specify; e.g., muscle weakness, paralysis, balancing difficulties, coordination)
- Report of dizziness, vertigo, syncope

**Safety Factors**

- Smoking in bed or near oxygen
- Lack of safety precautions, safety education
- History of previous trauma, accidental injury (falling, car accidents)
- Entering unlighted rooms
- Use of cracked dishware or glasses
- Use of thin or worn potholders or mitts
- Driving mechanically unsafe vehicles; driving after consuming alcoholic beverages, drugs

*Continues*

### Risk for Injury (1978)—*cont'd*

+ Driving at excessive speeds or without necessary visual aids
+ Nonuse or misuse of seat restraints, headgear for cyclists and passengers
+ Overexposure to sun or sun lamps

#### Child Supervision

+ Bathing in very hot water; unsupervised bathing of young children
+ Experimenting with chemicals or gasoline; contact with acid or alkali
+ Play or work near vehicle pathways (driveways, roads, railroad tracks)
+ Children playing with matches, candles, cigarettes, fireworks, gunpowder, sharp-edged toys
+ Children riding in front seat of automobile; unrestrained babies riding in car
+ Children playing without gates at top of stairs
+ Highly flammable children's toys or clothing

#### Environment

+ Sliding on coarse bed linen and struggling within bed restraints
+ High beds
+ Slippery, littered, or obstructed floors, stairs, walkways (wet, highly waxed, snow, ice)
+ Unanchored rugs, unsturdy or absent stair rails; unsteady ladders or chairs
+ Bathtub without hand grips or anti-slip equipment
+ Unanchored electric wires
+ Knives stored uncovered
+ Guns or ammunition stored in unlocked area
+ Large icicles hanging from roof

- Overloaded fuse boxes or electrical outlets; faulty electrical plugs, frayed wires; defective appliances
- Pot handles facing toward front of stove
- Potential igniting gas leaks; delayed lighting of fast burner or oven; grease waste collected on stoves
- High-crime neighborhood, unsafe roads, or road-crossing conditions
- Exposure to dangerous machinery, contact with rapidly moving machinery, industrial belts, pulleys
- Inadequately stored combustible or corrosive materials (matches, oily rags, lye)
- Unsafe window protection in homes with young children
- Insufficient finances to purchase safety equipment or make repairs

## OUTCOME

### Physical Injury

- Absence of injuries from accidents and trauma

## Risk for Vascular Trauma  (2008)

**DEFINITION**

At risk for damage to a vein and its surrounding tissues related to the presence of a catheter and/or infused solutions

**RISK FACTORS**

- Lack of understanding of site, catheter, and/or infusion*
- Catheter type
- Catheter width
- Impaired ability to visualize the insertion site
- Inadequate catheter fixation
- Infusion rate
- Insertion site
- Length of insertion time
- Nature of solution (e.g., concentration, chemical irritant, temperature, pH)

**OUTCOME**

**Health Management**

- Absence of trauma to insertion site

*Characteristic added to broaden application of concept to home infusions and self-management.

## Risk for Bleeding  (2008)

### DEFINITION

At risk for loss/decrease in blood volume that may compromise health

### RISK FACTORS

- Aneurysm
- Circumcision
- Deficient knowledge
- Disseminated intravascular coagulopathy
- History of falls
- Gastrointestinal disorders (e.g., gastric ulcer disease, polyps, varices)
- Impaired liver function (e.g., cirrhosis, hepatitis)
- Inherent coagulopathies (e.g., thrombocytopenia)
- Postpartum complications (e.g., uterine atony, retained placenta)
- Pregnancy-related complications (e.g., placenta previa, molar pregnancy, abruption pregnancy)
- Trauma
- Treatment-related side effects (e.g., surgery, medications, administration of platelet deficient blood products, chemotherapy)

### OUTCOME

- Intact vascular system
- Uses precautions to avoid trauma

## Risk for Falls (2000)

**DEFINITION**

Increased susceptibility for falling that may cause physical harm

**RISK FACTORS**

**General Factors: Children**

- Less than 2 years of age
- Male gender when less than 1 year of age
- Lack of auto restraints
- Lack of gate on stairs and window guards
- Bed located near window
- Unattended infant on bed, changing table, or sofa
- Lack of parental supervision

**General Factors: Adult**

- History of falls
- Wheelchair use
- Age 65 or over
- Female (if older)
- Lives alone
- Lower limb prosthesis, assistive devices (e.g., walker, cane)

**Physiological Factors**

- Presence of acute illness
- Postoperative conditions
- Visual or hearing difficulties
- Arthritis
- Orthostatic hypotension
- Sleeplessness
- Feeling faint when turning or extending neck
- Anemia, Vascular Disease

# HEALTH-PERCEPTION–HEALTH-MANAGEMENT PATTERN

- Postprandial blood sugar change
- Diarrhea
- Decreased lower-extremity strength
- Foot problems (e.g., neuropathy)
- Impaired physical mobility and balance
- Gait disturbance
- Proprioceptive deficits (e.g., unilateral neglect)

## Cognitive Factors

- Diminished mental status (e.g., confusion, delirium, impaired reality testing)

## Chemical Factors

- Antihypertensive agents, diuretics (ACE inhibitors)
- Tricyclic antidepressants, antianxiety agents, hypnotics, tranquilizers
- Alcohol use
- Narcotics

## Environmental Factors

- Restraints
- Weather conditions (e.g., ice, wet floors)
- Throw/scatter rugs
- Cluttered environment
- Unfamiliar dimly lit room
- No anti-slip material in bathroom and shower

## OUTCOME

### Falls Occurrence

- No falls in the past _____ (define period of time)

## Risk for Perioperative Positioning Injury (1994)

**DEFINITION**

Presence of risk factors for injury as a result of the environmental conditions found in the perioperative setting

**RISK FACTORS**

- Sensory/perceptual disturbances caused by anesthesia
- Disorientation
- Immobilization
- Muscle weakness
- Obesity
- Emaciation
- Edema

**OUTCOME**

**Injury Control**

- Absence of perioperative injury

## Risk for Poisoning (1980)

### DEFINITION

Presence of risk factors for accidental exposure to (or ingestion of) drugs or dangerous products in doses sufficient to cause poisoning.

### RISK FACTORS

#### Environmental Factors

- Flaking, peeling paint or plaster in presence of young children
- Dangerous products placed or stored within reach of children or confused persons
- Medicines stored in unlocked cabinets accessible to children or confused persons
- Large supplies of drugs in the house
- Availability of illicit drug potentially contaminated by poisonous additives
- Chemical contamination of food or water
- Unprotected contact with heavy metals or chemicals
- Paint, lacquer, and so forth in poorly ventilated areas or without effective protection
- Presence of poisonous vegetation
- Presence of atmospheric pollution

#### Personal Factors

- Reduced vision
- Cognitive impairment or emotional difficulties
- Occupational setting without adequate safeguards
- Lack of safety or drug education
- Insufficient finances

*Continues*

**Risk for Poisoning  (1980)—*cont'd***

**OUTCOME**

**Personal Safety Behavior**

- Personal actions taken to prevent poisoning; absence of poisoning

## Risk for Suffocation (1980)

### DEFINITION

Presence of risk factors for accidental interruption in air available for inhalation

### RISK FACTORS

#### Personal Factors

- Reduced olfactory sensation
- Cognitive impairment or emotional difficulties
- Mobility impairment (bed mobility or ambulation)
- Knowledge deficit (safety education)
- Eating large mouthfuls of food

#### Safety Factors

- Vehicle warming in a closed garage
- Pillow placed in an infant's crib
- Propped bottle placed in an infant's crib
- Pacifier hung around an infant's neck
- Children playing in plastic bags, inserting small objects into their mouths or noses
- Discarded or unused refrigerators or freezers without removed doors
- Children left unattended in bathtubs or pools
- Household gas leaks
- Use of fuel-burning heaters not vented to the outside

### OUTCOME

#### Respiratory Status: Ventilation

- Movement of air in and out of lungs

## Ineffective Protection (Specify) (1990)

### DEFINITION

Decreased ability to guard self from internal or external threats such as illness or injury

### DEFINING CHARACTERISTICS

#### Diagnostic Cues

One or more of the following:

- ◆ Deficient immunity
- ◆ Impaired healing
- ◆ Altered clotting
- ◆ Maladaptive stress response
- ◆ Neurosensory alterations; disorientation

#### Supporting Cues

- ◆ Chilling, perspiring
- ◆ Dyspnea, cough
- ◆ Itching
- ◆ Restlessness
- ◆ Insomnia, fatigue, anorexia, weakness
- ◆ Immobility
- ◆ Pressure ulcers

### OUTCOME

#### Health-Promoting Behavior

- ◆ Personal actions taken to sustain or increase wellness

### ETIOLOGICAL OR RELATED FACTORS

- ◆ Alcohol abuse
- ◆ Inadequate nutrition

## HIGH-RISK POPULATIONS

- Abnormal blood profiles (leukopenia, thrombocytopenia, anemia, coagulation)
- Drug therapies (antineoplastic, corticosteroid, immune, anticoagulant, thrombolytic)
- Treatments (surgery, radiation, cancer, immune disorders)

## Disturbed Energy Field  (1994, 2004)

### DEFINITION

Disruption of the flow of energy surrounding a person's being that results in a disharmony of the body, mind, and/or spirit

### DEFINING CHARACTERISTICS

- ♦ Perceptions of changes in patterns of energy flow such as
  a. Movement (wave, spike, tingling, dense, flowing)
  b. Sounds (tone/words)
  c. Temperature change (warmth/coolness)
  d. Disruption of the field (deficit, vacant/hole/spike/bulge, obstruction, congestion, diminished flow in energy field)
  e. Visual changes (image/color)

### OUTCOME

#### Personal Health Status

- ♦ Overall physical, psychological, social, spiritual functioning meets norms for age

### ETIOLOGICAL OR RELATED FACTORS

Slowing or blocking of energy flows secondary to one or more of the following:

#### Pathophysiologic Factors

- ♦ Illness
- ♦ Pregnancy
- ♦ Injury

# HEALTH-PERCEPTION–HEALTH-MANAGEMENT PATTERN

## Treatment-Related Factors

- Immobility
- Labor and delivery
- Perioperative experience
- Chemotherapy

## Situational Factors

- Pain
- Fear
- Anxiety
- Grieving

## Maturational Factors

- Age-related developmental crises

## NOTES

**NOTES**

## NOTES

# Nutritional–Metabolic Pattern

## Imbalanced Nutrition: More Than Body Requirements or Exogenous Obesity (1975, 2000)

### DEFINITION
Intake of nutrients exceeds metabolic need.

### DEFINING CHARACTERISTICS
#### Diagnostic Cues

- Triceps skin fold greater than 15 mm in men and 25 mm in women
- Body mass index 30 or higher (obesity); 25 or more (overweight)
- Weight greater than 20% over ideal for height and frame (obesity); weight 10% to 20% over ideal for height and frame (overweight)
- Reported intake greater than recommended daily allowance

#### Supporting Cues

- Pale conjunctiva and mucous membranes

### OUTCOME
#### Nutritional Status: Nutrient Intake

- Adequate pattern of nutrient intake for metabolic need

#### Weight: Body Mass

- Body weight, muscle, and fat are congruent with recommendations for height, frame, gender and age

### ETIOLOGICAL OR RELATED FACTORS

- Food intake–energy expenditure imbalance
- Dysfunctional eating patterns (reported or observed)
- Pairing food with other activities

## NUTRITIONAL–METABOLIC PATTERN

- Concentrating food intake at end of day
- Eating in response to external cues (time of day, social situation)
- Eating in response to internal cues other than hunger (anxiety, depression)
- Sedentary activity level (relative to caloric intake)
- Knowledge deficit (nutritional requirements)

## HIGH-RISK POPULATIONS

- History of childhood obesity/overweight
- Emotional disorders, life stress
- Enforced sedentary lifestyle (e.g., wheelchair bound)

**Imbalanced Nutrition: Risk for More Than Body Requirements or *Risk for Obesity* (1975, 2000)**

### DEFINITION

Presence of risk factors for intake that exceeds metabolic need

### RISK FACTORS

- Dysfunctional eating patterns
- Pairing food with other activities
- Concentrating food intake at end of day
- Eating in response to external cues (time of day, social situation)
- Eating in response to internal cues (anxiety, depression)
- Sedentary activity level
- Reported or observed obesity in one or both parents; hereditary predisposition
- Rapid transition across growth percentiles in infants or children
- Excessive intake relative to energy expenditure during late gestational life, early infancy, and adolescence
- Dysfunctional psychological conditioning in response to food (use of food as reward or comfort measure)
- Frequent, closely spaced pregnancies; reported or observed higher baseline at beginning of pregnancy
- Low financial resources (selection of lower cost, high-caloric foods)

### OUTCOME

### Weight: Body Mass

- Body weight, muscle, and fat are congruent with recommendations for height, frame, gender, and age

> **Imbalanced Nutrition: Less Than Body Requirements or Nutritional Deficit (Specify Type) (1975, 2000)**

## DEFINITION

Insufficient intake of nutrients to meet metabolic needs

## DEFINING CHARACTERISTICS

### Diagnostic Cues

- Body mass index 18 or less
- Weight loss (with or without adequate intake), 20% or more under ideal body weight
- Reported or observed food intake less than recommended minimum daily requirement

### Supporting Cues

- Fatigue
- Capillary fragility
- Pale conjunctiva and mucous membranes
- Excessive hair loss, poor muscle tone
- Hyperactive bowel sounds, abdominal cramping, pain
- Diarrhea and/or steatorrhea

## OUTCOME

### Nutritional Status: Nutrient Intake

- Adequate pattern of nutrient intake for metabolic need

### Weight: Body Mass

- Body weight, muscle, and fat are congruent with recommendations for height, frame, gender, and age

*Continues*

**Imbalanced Nutrition: Less Than Body Requirements or Nutritional Deficit (Specify Type) (1975, 2000)—*cont'd***

## ETIOLOGICAL OR RELATED FACTORS

+ Buccal cavity discomfort or pain
+ Pain with mastication (dental caries)
+ Altered or loss of taste sensation
+ Inability to prepare or obtain food
+ Diarrhea, steatorrhea
+ Knowledge deficit (daily requirements)
+ Financial limitations
+ Social isolation
+ Anorexia, setophobia, early satiety
+ Chemical dependency
+ Emotional stress
+ Food faddism, dieting practices
+ Muscle weakness (mastication, swallowing)

## HIGH-RISK POPULATIONS

+ Hypermetabolic or catabolic states
+ Absorptive disorders
+ Low income

## Readiness for Enhanced Nutrition (2002)

### DEFINITION

Pattern of nutrient intake that is sufficient for meeting metabolic needs and can be strengthened

### DEFINING CHARACTERISTICS

- ♦ Expresses desire/willingness to enhance nutrition
- ♦ Eats regularly
- ♦ Consumes adequate food and fluid
- ♦ Expresses knowledge of health food and fluid choices
- ♦ Follows an appropriate standard for types of intake (e.g., food pyramid, Diabetic Association Guidelines)
- ♦ Prepares and stores food and fluids safely
- ♦ Attitude toward eating and drinking is congruent with health goals

### OUTCOME

### Nutritional Status: Nutrient Intake

- ♦ Adequate pattern of nutrient intake for metabolic need

### Adult Failure to Thrive* (1998)

#### DEFINITION

Progressive functional deterioration of a physical and cognitive nature (associated with multisystem disease that is no longer responsive to medical interventions; condition may respond to psychosocial nursing interventions when diagnosed early)

#### DEFINING CHARACTERISTICS

- Anorexia (loss of appetite); does not eat meals when offered; states does not have an appetite, not hungry, or "I don't want to eat"
- Inadequate nutritional intake. Eating less than body requirements; consumes minimal to none of food at most meals (i.e., consumes less than 75% of normal requirements at each, or most, meals)
- Weight loss (decreased body mass from baseline weight, i.e., 5% unintentional weight loss in 1 month, 10% unintentional weight loss in 6 months)
- Physical decline (decline in bodily function with evidence of fatigue, dehydration, incontinence of bowel and bladder; frequent exacerbation of chronic health problems such as congestive heart failure, pneumonia, and urinary tract infections)
- Cognitive decline (decline in mental processing, as evidenced by problems with responding appropriately to environmental stimuli, demonstrates difficulty in reasoning, decision making, judgment, memory and concentration, decreased perception)
- Decreased social skills/social withdrawal (noticeable decrease in attempts to form or participate in cooperative and interdependent relationships, e.g.,

*This diagnosis meets the criteria for a syndrome.

decreased verbal communication with staff, family, friends; decreased participation in activities of daily living and activities that the person once enjoyed)

♦ Self-care deficit (e.g., no longer looks after or takes charge of physical cleanliness or appearance; difficulty performing simple self-care tasks; neglects home environment and/or financial responsibilities; apathy, as evidenced by lack of observable feeling or emotion in terms of normal activities of daily living and environment)

♦ Depression (altered mood state): expresses feeling "depressed"

and/or one or more of the following:

♦ Feelings of sadness, low in spirits and mood

♦ Loss of interest in pleasurable outlets such as food, sex, work, friends, family, hobbies, or entertainment

♦ Apathy, lethargy, fatigue

♦ Decreased motivation in performing activities of daily living

♦ Appears depressed (e.g., spends much of the time in bed with face to wall), verbalizes desire for death

♦ Helplessness

## OUTCOME

### Will to Live

♦ Presence of desire, determination, and effort to thrive

## HIGH-RISK POPULATIONS

♦ Primarily seen in adult/older persons (1) who have multisystem disease that is no longer responsive to medical interventions (2) who are coping with the ensuing problems, and (3) who have a remarkably diminished ability to manage own care

## Ineffective Breastfeeding   (1988)

### DEFINITION

Dissatisfaction or difficulty with the breastfeeding process experienced by mother or infant/child

### DEFINING CHARACTERISTICS

#### Diagnostic Cues

Report or observation of one or more of the following behavioral patterns:

+ Actual or perceived inadequate milk supply
+ Infant inability to attach to maternal breast correctly
+ No observable signs of oxytocin release
+ Observable signs of inadequate infant intake
+ Nonsustained or insufficient opportunity for suckling at the breast
+ Insufficient emptying of each breast per feeding
+ Persistence of sore nipples beyond the first week of breastfeeding
+ Infant exhibiting fussiness and crying within first hour after breastfeeding; unresponsive to comfort measures
+ Infant arching and crying at the breast; infant resisting latching on

#### Supporting Cues

+ Previous history of breastfeeding failure
+ Report of unsatisfactory breastfeeding process

### OUTCOME

#### Breastfeeding Establishment: Infant

+ Infant attachment to and sucking from the mother's breast for nourishment during the first 3 weeks of breastfeeding

# NUTRITIONAL–METABOLIC PATTERN

## Breastfeeding Establishment: Maternal

♦ Maternal establishment of proper attachment of an infant to, and sucking from, the breast for nourishment during the first 3 weeks of breastfeeding

## ETIOLOGICAL OR RELATED FACTORS

♦ Knowledge deficit (breastfeeding)
♦ Interrupted breastfeeding
♦ Maternal anxiety; maternal ambivalence
♦ Prematurity or infant anomaly
♦ Maternal breast anomaly; previous breast surgery
♦ Infant supplemental feedings with artificial nipple
♦ Poor infant sucking reflex
♦ Nonsupportive partner or family

## HIGH-RISK POPULATIONS

♦ Previous history of breastfeeding failure
♦ Infant anomaly

## Interrupted Breastfeeding (1992)

### DEFINITION
Break in continuity of breastfeeding process as a result of inability or inadvisability to put baby to breast for feeding

### DEFINING CHARACTERISTICS
#### Diagnostic Cues
+ Infant does not receive nourishment at the breast for some or all feedings
+ Presence of factors interfering with maternal desire to maintain lactation and provide (or eventually provide) her breast milk for infant's nutritional needs (specify)

### OUTCOME
#### Breastfeeding Maintenance
+ Continuation of breastfeeding for nourishment of an infant/toddler

### ETIOLOGICAL OR RELATED FACTORS
+ Knowledge deficit (expression and storage of breast milk)
+ Mother–infant separation (e.g., maternal employment)
+ Contraindications to breastfeeding (e.g., drugs, true breast milk jaundice)
+ Need to abruptly wean infant (e.g., maternal or infant illness)

### HIGH-RISK POPULATIONS
+ Prematurity

## Effective Breastfeeding* (1990)

### DEFINITION
Mother–infant dyad/family exhibits adequate proficiency and
satisfaction with breastfeeding process

### DEFINING CHARACTERISTICS
#### Diagnostic Cues
- Mother able to position infant at breast to promote a
  successful latch-on response
- Infant is content after feeding
- Appropriate infant weight patterns for age
- Regular and sustained suckling/swallowing at the
  breast
- Effective mother–infant communication patterns
  (infant cues; maternal interpretation and response)

#### Supporting Cues
- Signs or symptoms of oxytocin release (let-down or
  milk ejection reflex)
- Adequate infant elimination patterns for age
- Eagerness of infant to nurse
- Maternal verbalization of satisfaction with the
  breastfeeding process
- Basic breastfeeding knowledge
- Normal breast structure
- Normal infant oral structure
- Infant gestational age greater than 34 weeks
- Presence of support sources
- Maternal confidence

*Continues*

*This diagnostic category does not represent a problem or risk. As with other
healthy states or processes, periodic assessment is advisable.

## Effective Breastfeeding (1990)—*cont'd*

**OUTCOME**

**Breastfeeding Establishment: Infant**

♦ Infant attachment to and sucking from the mother's breast for nourishment during the first 3 weeks of breastfeeding

**Breastfeeding Establishment: Maternal**

♦ Maternal establishment of proper attachment of an infant to and sucking from the breast for nourishment during the first 3 weeks of breastfeeding

## Ineffective Infant Feeding Pattern* (1992)

### DEFINITION

Impaired ability to suck or coordinate the suck-swallow response

### DEFINING CHARACTERISTICS

#### Diagnostic Cues

- ♦ Inability to initiate or sustain an effective suck
- ♦ Inability to coordinate sucking, swallowing, and breathing

### HIGH-RISK POPULATIONS

- ♦ Prematurity
- ♦ Neurological impairment/delay (specify)
- ♦ Prolonged nothing by mouth
- ♦ Anatomic abnormality (specify e.g., cleft lip, cleft palate)
- ♦ Oral hypersensitivity

### OUTCOME

#### Breastfeeding Establishment: Infant

- ♦ Infant attachment to and sucking from the mother's breast for nourishment during the first 3 weeks of breastfeeding

---

*This condition is frequently a focus for intervention (i.e., an etiological/related factor).

## Neonatal Jaundice* (2008)

### DEFINITION

Yellow-orange tint of the neonate's skin and mucous membranes that occurs after 24 hours of life as a result of unconjugated bilirubin in the circulation

### DEFINING CHARACTERISTICS
#### Diagnostic Cues

+ Neonate age 1–7 days
+ Abnormal blood profile (hemolysis, total serum bilirubin > 2 mg/d.; total serum bilirubin in high risk range for age in hour-specific nomogram)
+ Yellow-orange skin
+ Yellow sclera

#### Supporting Cues

+ Abnormal weight loss (> 7% to 8% in breastfeeding newborn; 15% in term infant)
+ Feeding pattern not well established
+ Infant experiences difficulty in making transition to extrauterine life
+ Stool passage delayed

### ETIOLOGICAL OR RELATED FACTORS

+ None specified

### OUTCOME
#### Skin Status

+ Skin normal color

---

*May be physiological or pathological with a genetic base. Refer for medical evaluation if diagnosed.

# NUTRITIONAL–METABOLIC PATTERN

## OUTCOME

## Tissue Integrity: Skin and Mucous Membrane

- ♦ Structural intactness and normal physiological functions of skin and mucous membrane

## ETIOLOGICAL OR RELATED FACTORS

- ♦ Ineffective oral hygiene practices
- ♦ Chemical irritants (e.g., alcohol, tobacco, acidic foods, regular use of inhalers)
- ♦ Dehydration (excessive fluid loss, e.g., sweating, vomiting)
- ♦ Mouth breathing
- ♦ Malnutrition or vitamin deficiency
- ♦ Stress, depression
- ♦ Immunocompromised
- ♦ Medication side effects
- ♦ Lack of or decreased salivation
- ♦ Barriers to oral self-care
- ♦ Barriers to professional care
- ♦ Poorly fitting dental prostheses
- ♦ Mechanical factors: tubes (endotracheal/nasogastric), ill-fitting dentures, braces, biting/chewing

## HIGH-RISK POPULATIONS

- ♦ Oral surgery, trauma
- ♦ Cleft lip or palate
- ♦ Radiation therapy (head/neck/mouth) or chemotherapy
- ♦ Pathology (e.g., cancer, infection, periodontal disease, decreased platelets)
- ♦ Loss of supportive oral structures
- ♦ Aging-related loss of connective, adipose, or bone tissue
- ♦ Diminished hormone levels (women)

## Impaired Dentition (1998)

### DEFINITION

Disruption in tooth development/eruption patterns or structural integrity of individual teeth

### DEFINING CHARACTERISTICS

- Missing or loose teeth or complete absence of teeth
- Toothache
- Sensitivity to heat or cold
- Excessive plaque
- Crown or root caries
- Halitosis
- Tooth enamel discoloration
- Excessive calculus
- Worn down or abraded teeth
- Tooth fracture(s)
- Erosion of enamel
- Asymmetrical facial expression
- Incomplete eruption for age (primary or permanent teeth)
- Malocclusion or tooth misalignment
- Premature loss of primary teeth

### OUTCOME

#### Oral Hygiene

- Development and integrity of teeth sufficient for chewing and mastication of food

### ETIOLOGICAL OR RELATED FACTORS

- Ineffective oral hygiene
- Barriers to self-care (specify)
- Access or economic barriers to professional care
- Nutritional deficits, dietary habits

## NUTRITIONAL–METABOLIC PATTERN

- Premature loss of primary teeth
- Excessive intake of fluorides
- Chronic vomiting
- Chronic use of tobacco, coffee or tea, red wine
- Knowledge deficit (dental health)
- Excessive use of abrasive cleaning agents; bruxism

## Deficient Fluid Volume* (1978, 1996)

### DEFINITION

Decreased intravascular, interstitial, and/or intracellular fluid below normal range for individual (this refers to dehydration—water loss alone without change in sodium)

### DEFINING CHARACTERISTICS

- ♦ Thirst
- ♦ Sudden weight loss (except in third spacing)
- ♦ Decreased blood pressure
- ♦ Increased pulse rate
- ♦ Decreased urine output (oliguria)
- ♦ Increased urine concentration, increased specific gravity
- ♦ Increased body temperature
- ♦ Decreased pulse volume or pressure
- ♦ Change in mental state
- ♦ Dry skin and mucous membranes
- ♦ Decreased skin turgor
- ♦ Weakness
- ♦ Decreased venous filling
- ♦ Elevated hematocrit

### OUTCOME

#### Fluid Balance

- ♦ Balance in the intracellular and extracellular compartments of the body

### ETIOLOGICAL OR RELATED FACTORS

- ♦ Active fluid volume loss (normal routes, tubes; diarrhea)
- ♦ Failure of regulatory mechanisms

*If diagnosed, refer for medical evaluation.

## HIGH-RISK POPULATIONS

- Conditions affecting access to fluids
- Conditions affecting absorption of fluids
- Hypermetabolic states (hyperthermia, etc.)
- Extremes of age/weight

### Risk for Deficient Fluid Volume  (1978)

**DEFINITION**

Presence of risk factors for decrease in body fluid (vascular, cellular, or intracellular dehydration)

**RISK FACTORS**

- Impaired ability to take in fluids
- Excessive loss of fluid through normal routes (describe; e.g., diarrhea)
- Loss of fluid through abnormal routes (describe; e.g., indwelling tubes)
- Excessive insensible loss
- Deviations affecting access to fluids, intake of fluids, or absorption of fluids (e.g., physical immobility, unconsciousness)
- Medications (e.g., diuretics)
- Factors influencing fluid requirements (e.g., hypermetabolic states; hyperthermia; dry, hot environment)
- Extremes of age
- Hyperthermia
- Knowledge deficit (fluid volume needs)
- Increased fluid output
- Urinary frequency
- Weight extremes

**OUTCOME**

**Fluid Balance**

- Balance in the intracellular and extracellular compartments of the body

**Hydration**

- Adequate water in the intracellular and extracellular compartments of the body

## Excess Fluid Volume* (1982, 1996)

### DEFINITION

Increased isotonic fluid retention

### DEFINING CHARACTERISTICS

- ♦ Weight gain over short period
- ♦ Intake exceeds output
- ♦ Altered electrolytes
- ♦ Increased central venous pressure
- ♦ Third heart sound (S3 gallop)
- ♦ Blood pressure changes
- ♦ Abnormal breath sounds (rales or crackles)
- ♦ Dyspnea (shortness of breath), orthopnea
- ♦ Pleural effusion
- ♦ Pulmonary congestion, pulmonary artery pressure changes
- ♦ Hepatic congestion, positive hepatojugular reflex
- ♦ Anasarca, oliguria, specific gravity changes
- ♦ Decreased blood urea nitrogen; azotemia
- ♦ Decreased hemoglobin and hematocrit
- ♦ Central venous pressure 11 cm water
- ♦ Change in mental status (restlessness)

### OUTCOME

#### Fluid Balance

- ♦ Water balance in the intracellular and extracellular compartments of the body

*Continues*

*If diagnosed, refer for medical evaluation.

**Excess Fluid Volume  (1982, 1996)—*cont'd***

### ETIOLOGICAL OR RELATED FACTORS

- Excess sodium intake (e.g., excess isotonic intravenous fluids)
- Excess fluid intake
- Compromised regulatory mechanism

### HIGH-RISK POPULATIONS

- Renal failure
- Congestive heart failure
- Cirrhosis
- Cushing's syndrome

## Risk for Imbalanced Fluid Volume (1998)

### DEFINITION
Risk for decrease, increase, or rapid shift among intravascular, interstitial, and/or intracellular fluid compartments

### RISK FACTORS
- Major invasive procedure
- Abdominal surgery
- Ascites
- Pancreatitis
- Burns
- Receiving apheresis
- Intestinal obstruction
- Sepsis
- Traumatic injury (e.g., fractured hip)

### OUTCOME
### Fluid Balance
- Water balanced in the intracellular and extracellular compartments of the body

## Readiness for Enhanced Fluid Balance (2002)

### DEFINITION

Pattern of equilibrium between fluid volume and chemical composition of body fluids that is sufficient for meeting physical needs and can be strengthened.

### DEFINING CHARACTERISTICS

- Expresses desire/willingness to enhance fluid balance
- Stable weight
- Fluid intake meets daily need; no excessive thirst
- Straw-colored urine
- Specific gravity within normal limits
- Moist mucous membranes
- Good tissue turgor
- Urine output appropriate for intake
- No evidence of edema or dehydration

### OUTCOME

### Fluid Balance

- Water balanced in the intracellular and extracellular compartments of the body.

## Risk for Electrolyte Imbalance (2008)

**DEFINITION**

At risk for change in serum electrolyte levels that may compromise health

**RISK FACTORS**

- Diarrhea
- Endocrine dysfunction
- Fluid imbalance (e.g., dehydration, water intoxication)
- Impaired regulatory mechanisms (e.g., diabetes insipidus, syndrome of inappropriate secretion of antidiuretic hormone)
- Renal dysfunction
- Treatment-related side effects (e.g., medications, drains)
- Vomiting

**OUTCOME**

**Electrolyte Balance**

- Serum electrolyte balance

## NUTRITIONAL–METABOLIC PATTERN

### Impaired Skin Integrity* (1975, 1998)

### DEFINITION

Break in dermis and/or epidermis (see also Pressure Ulcer)

### DEFINING CHARACTERISTICS

#### Diagnostic Cues

- ◆ Disruption of skin surface (epidermis)
- ◆ Destruction of skin layers (dermis)
- ◆ Invasion of body structures (deep ulceration)

### OUTCOME

#### Tissue Integrity: Skin and Mucous Membranes

- ◆ Structural intactness and normal physiological function of skin and mucous membranes

### ETIOLOGICAL OR RELATED FACTORS

- ◆ Altered circulation, metabolic state
- ◆ Hyperthermia or hypothermia
- ◆ Humidity
- ◆ Alteration in turgor (elasticity)
- ◆ Altered nutritional status (obesity, emaciation)
- ◆ Altered pigmentation
- ◆ Developmental factors; psychogenic factors

### HIGH-RISK POPULATIONS

- ◆ Physical immobilization
- ◆ Sensory-motor loss (cerebrovascular accident, spinal cord injury)
- ◆ Loss of consciousness
- ◆ Obesity
- ◆ Emaciation
- ◆ Immunological deficit
- ◆ Radiation

*See also Pressure Ulcer, Stage II–IV.

### Risk for Impaired Skin Integrity or Risk for Skin Breakdown* (1975, 1998)

#### DEFINITION

Presence of risk factors for skin ulceration/excoriation; use a risk assessment tool (e.g., Braden Scale) to determine risk

#### RISK FACTORS

+ Unable to shift position at least every 1.5 to 2 hours (impaired mobility; immobilization)
+ Reddened skin area (altered tissue perfusion), especially over bony prominences
+ Verbalized pain or discomfort in local area, especially over bony prominences (possible deep-tissue damage)
+ Presence of shearing forces, pressure (restraints, sustained pressure from casts), friction
+ Nutritional deficit (e.g., protein, ascorbic acid deficiency)
+ Excretions/secretions on skin
+ Skeletal prominence
+ Altered skin turgor (change in elasticity)
+ Altered sensation, cognitive impairment (e.g., decreased consciousness)
+ Altered metabolic state, anemia
+ Altered circulation, edema, arteriosclerosis
+ Psychogenic factors
+ High humidity, environmental temperature
+ Hypothermia or hyperthermia
+ Medication (producing cellular breakdown)
+ Altered pigmentation
+ Decreased fatty tissue, skeletal prominence
+ Immunologic factors

*Continues*

*See also Pressure Ulcer Stage I.

## Risk for Impaired Skin Integrity or Risk for Skin Breakdown (1975, 1998)—*cont'd*

- ♦ Chemical substances on skin
- ♦ Radiation

**OUTCOME**

**Tissue Integrity: Skin and Mucous Membranes**

- ♦ Structural intactness and normal physiological function of skin and mucous membranes

## Pressure Ulcer (Specify Stage)*

### DEFINITION

Break in skin integrity, usually over bony prominences, associated with lying or sitting for prolonged periods (specify stage)

### DEFINING CHARACTERISTICS

#### Diagnostic Cues

+ Ulceration (disruption of skin surface, destruction of skin layers usually over bony prominences)

and/or

+ Verbalization of pain, discomfort, or numbness over bony prominence *without* exterior skin destruction (deep decubitus)

| | |
|---|---|
| **Stage I:** | Reddened area; no break in skin. (Non-blanchable erythema of intact skin. Note that reactive hyperemia can normally be expected to be present for 1D 2 to 3D 4 as long as the pressure occluded blood flow to the area. This should not be confused with stage I pressure ulcer.) |
| **Stage II:** | Reddened area; small ulceration. (Partial-thickness skin loss involving epidermis and/or dermis. The ulcer is superficial and appears clinically as an abrasion, blister, or shallow crater.) |

*Continues*

---

*Clinical Practice Guideline 3: *Pressure Ulcers in Adults: Prediction and Prevention.* Rockville, MD: USDHHS, Agency for Health Care Policy and Research; 1992. See this for detection, prevention, diagnosis, and treatment guidelines. Refer for medical evaluation if unresponsive to nursing measures and particularly if progression continues to stage III or stage IV.

### Pressure Ulcer (Specify Stage)—*cont'd*

**Stage III:**   Deep ulceration with drainage; no necrosis. (Full-thickness skin loss involving damage to or necrosis of subcutaneous tissue that may extend down to, but not through, fascia. The ulcer appears clinically as a deep crater with or without undermining of adjacent tissue.)

**Stage IV:**   Deep ulceration; necrotic area. (Full-thickness skin loss with extensive destruction, tissue necrosis or damage to muscle, bone, or supporting structures, and/or tendon or joint capsule. Note that undermining and sinus tracts may also be associated with stage IV pressure ulcers.)

## OUTCOME

### Tissue Integrity: Skin

♦ Structural intactness and normal physiological function of skin

## ETIOLOGICAL OR RELATED FACTORS

♦ Prolonged pressure
♦ Friction, shear injury
♦ Immobility
♦ Incontinence
♦ Undernutrition (protein, vitamin C)
♦ Sensory-motor loss
♦ Cognitive impairment

## HIGH-RISK POPULATIONS

♦ Hemiplegia, quadriplegia, hemiparesis (e.g., cerebral vascular accident (stroke), spinal cord injury)
♦ Orthopedic problems with immobilization (e.g., femoral fracture)
♦ Bed rest (e.g., critical care)

## Impaired Tissue Integrity (Specify Type) (1986, 1998)

### DEFINITION

Damage to mucous membrane or to corneal, integumentary, or subcutaneous tissue (specify type of tissue and impairment).

### DEFINING CHARACTERISTICS

- Damaged or destroyed tissue (cornea, mucous membrane, integumentary, or subcutaneous)

### OUTCOME

### Tissue Integrity: Skin and Mucous Membranes

- Structural intactness and normal physiological function of skin and mucous membranes

### ETIOLOGICAL OR RELATED FACTORS

- Altered circulation
- Nutritional deficit or excess
- Fluid deficit or excess
- Knowledge deficit
- Impaired physical mobility
- Irritants
  - Chemical (body excretions, secretions, medications)
  - Thermal (temperature extremes)
  - Mechanical (pressure, shear, friction)
  - Radiation (including therapeutic radiation)

## Latex Allergy Response (1998)

### DEFINITION

Allergic response to natural latex rubber products

### DEFINING CHARACTERISTICS
#### Type I Reaction

- Immediate reactions (< 1 hour) to latex proteins (can be life threatening)
- Contact urticaria progressing to generalized symptoms
- Edema of the lips, tongue, uvula, and/or throat
- Shortness of breath, tightness in chest, wheezing, bronchospasm leading to respiratory arrest
- Hypotension, syncope, cardiac arrest
- Facial itching
- Oral itching
- Gastrointestinal characteristics
  - Abdominal pain
  - Nausea
- Generalized characteristics
  - Flushing
  - General discomfort
  - Generalized edema
  - Increasing complaint of total body warmth
  - Restlessness

May also include

- Orofacial characteristics
  - Edema of sclera or eyelids
  - Erythema and/or itching of the eyes
  - Tearing of the eyes
  - Nasal congestion, itching, and/or erythema
  - Rhinorrhea
  - Facial erythema

- Facial, oral itching
- Abdominal pain, nausea
- Generalized symptoms
  - Flushing; increasing complaint of total body warmth
  - Generalized discomfort/generalized edema
  - Restless

## Type IV Reaction

- Eczema
- Irritation, redness, chapped or cracked skin or blisters
- Reaction to additives causes discomfort
  (e.g., thiurams, carbamates)
- Delayed onset (hours)
- No immune mechanism response

## OUTCOME

## Tissue Integrity: Skin and Mucous Membranes

- Structural intactness and normal physiological
  function of skin and mucous membranes

## Risk for Latex Allergy Response (1998)

### DEFINITION
Risk for allergic response to natural latex rubber products

### RISK FACTORS
- Multiple surgical procedures especially from infancy (e.g., spina bifida)
- Allergy to bananas, avocados, tropical fruits, kiwi, chestnuts
- Professions with daily exposure to latex (e.g., medicine, nursing, dentistry)
- Conditions needing continuous or intermittent catheterization
- History of reactions to latex (balloons, condoms, gloves)
- Allergies to poinsettia plants
- History of allergies and asthma

### OUTCOME
### Tissue Integrity: Skin and Mucous Membranes
- Structural intactness and normal physiological function of skin and mucous membranes

## Ineffective Thermoregulation (1986)

### DEFINITION

Temperature fluctuation between hypothermia
and hyperthermia

### DEFINING CHARACTERISTICS

#### Diagnostic Cues

- ♦ Fluctuations in body temperature above or below the
  normal range (see defining characteristics of
  Hypothermia and Hyperthermia)

### OUTCOME

#### Thermoregulation

- ♦ Balance among heat production, heat gain, and
  heat loss

### ETIOLOGICAL OR RELATED FACTORS

- ♦ Fluctuating environmental temperature

### HIGH-RISK POPULATIONS

- ♦ Trauma or illness influencing central regulation
- ♦ Extremes of age (prematurity, immaturity, very old)

## Hyperthermia (1986)

### DEFINITION
Body temperature elevated above normal range

### DEFINING CHARACTERISTICS
#### Diagnostic Cues
+ Increase in body temperature above normal range for age

#### Supporting Cues
+ Flushed skin
+ Skin warm to touch
+ Increased respiratory rate
+ Tachycardia
+ Seizures or convulsions (a consequence of hyperthermia)

### OUTCOME
#### Thermoregulation
+ Balance among heat production, heat gain, and heat loss resulting in normal temperature

### ETIOLOGICAL OR RELATED FACTORS
+ Exposure to hot environment
+ Vigorous activity
+ Medications/anesthesia
+ Inappropriate clothing
+ Increased metabolic rate
+ Illness or trauma
+ Dehydration
+ Inability or decreased ability to perspire

### Hypothermia (1986, 1988)

**DEFINITION**

Body temperature reduced below normal range

**DEFINING CHARACTERISTICS**

**Diagnostic Cues**

- Reduction in body temperature below normal range for age

**Supporting Cues**

- Shivering (mild)
- Cool skin; pallor (moderate); piloerection
- Slow capillary refill
- Tachycardia; cyanotic nail beds
- Hypertension

**OUTCOME**

**Thermoregulation**

- Balance among heat production, heat gain, and heat loss resulting in normal temperature

**ETIOLOGICAL OR RELATED FACTORS**

- Exposure to cool or cold environment
- Illness or trauma
- Inability or decreased ability to shiver
- Malnutrition, decreased metabolic rate, inactivity, aging
- Vasodilation, evaporation from skin in cool environment
- Damage to hypothalamus

## Risk for Imbalanced Body Temperature* (1986, 2000)

### DEFINITION
Presence of risk factors for failure to maintain body temperature within normal range

### RISK FACTORS
- Illness or trauma affecting temperature regulation
- Altered metabolic rate
- Dehydration
- Extremes of age
- Sedatives, anesthesia
- Medications causing vasoconstriction or vasodilation
- Exposure to cold/cool or warm/hot environments
- Inactivity or vigorous activity
- Inappropriate clothing for environmental temperature
- Extremes of weight

### OUTCOME
#### Thermoregulation
- Balance among heat production, heat gain, and heat loss resulting in normal temperature

#### Thermoregulation: Newborn
- Balance among heat production, heat gain, and heat loss during the first 28 days of life

*See also Ineffective Thermoregulation.

## Risk for Impaired Liver Function (2007)

**DEFINITION**

Risk for liver dysfunction

**RISK FACTORS**

- Hepatotoxic medications (e.g., acetaminophen, statins)
- HIV and co-occurring infection
- Substance abuse (e.g., alcohol, cocaine)
- Viral infection (e.g., hepatitis A, hepatitis B, hepatitis C, Epstein-Barr)

**OUTCOME**

- Functional liver metabolic processes

## Risk for Unstable Blood Glucose (2007)

### DEFINITION

Risk for variation of blood glucose (sugar) levels from the normal range

### RISK FACTORS

- Lack of diabetes management plan (e.g., action plan)
- Lack of adherence to diabetes management plan (e.g., action plan)
- Deficient knowledge of diabetes management (e.g., action plan)
- Dietary intake
- Inadequate blood glucose monitoring
- Medication management
- Lack of acceptance of diagnosis
- Developmental level
- Mental health status
- Physical activity level
- Physical health status
- Pregnancy
- Rapid growth periods
- Stress
- Weight gain or loss

### OUTCOME

### Blood Glucose Level

- Blood glucose level within normal range

## NOTES

## NOTES

# Elimination Pattern

## Constipation (1975, 1998)

### DEFINITION

Decrease in frequency of defecation accompanied by difficult or incomplete passage of hard, dry stool

### DEFINING CHARACTERISTICS

### Diagnostic Cues

- Bowel pattern: decreased frequency or volume
- Dry, hard, formed stool or unable to pass stool
- Reports feeling of rectal fullness or pressure

### Supporting Cues

- Straining with defecation
- Pain with defecation
- Abdominal tenderness with or without palpable muscle resistance; abdominal pain
- Distended abdomen; palpable rectal mass; palpable abdominal mass
- Increased abdominal pressure
- Abdominal dullness on percussion; borborygmi; hyperactive or hypoactive bowel sounds
- Severe flatus
- Presence of soft paste-like stool in rectum
- Anorexia, headache, indigestion; generalized fatigue
- Nausea, vomiting
- Bright red blood with stool
- Black or tarry stool

### Older Adults (Additional)

- Change in mental status
- Urinary incontinence
- Unexplained falls
- Elevated body temperature

# ELIMINATION PATTERN

## OUTCOME
### Bowel Elimination
- Formation and evacuation of stool

## ETIOLOGICAL OR RELATED FACTORS
### Functional
- Habitual denial/ignoring of urge to defecate
- Inadequate toileting (timeliness, positioning for defecation, privacy; irregular defecation habits)
- Insufficient physical activity
- Abdominal muscle weakness

### Psychological
- Depression
- Emotional stress
- Mental confusion

### Mechanical
- Obesity
- Hemorrhoids

## HIGH-RISK POPULATIONS
### Pharmacological
- Laxative overdose pattern
- Antilipemic agents
- Calcium carbonate; aluminum-containing antacids
- Nonsteroid anti-inflammatory agents
- Opiates, sedatives, antidepressants, phenothiazides
- Anticholinergics; bismuth salts
- Diuretics, sympathomimetics, calcium channel blockers

*Continues*

**Constipation (1975, 1998)—*cont'd***

**Mechanical**

- ◆ Rectal abscess or ulcer; anal fissures; tumors; anal stricture
- ◆ Pregnancy
- ◆ Megacolon (Hirschsprung's disease)
- ◆ Electrolyte imbalance
- ◆ Rectal prolapse
- ◆ Prostate enlargement
- ◆ Neurological impairment
- ◆ Retrocele
- ◆ Postsurgical obstruction

## Perceived Constipation  (1988)

### DEFINITION
Self-diagnosis of constipation and ensures daily bowel movement through abuse of laxatives, enemas, and/or suppositories

### DEFINING CHARACTERISTICS
### Diagnostic Cues
- Expectation of a daily bowel movement resulting in overuse of laxatives, enemas, and/or suppositories
- Expected passage of stool at same time every day

### OUTCOME
### Health Beliefs: Bowel Health
- Personal convictions consistent with bowel health

### ETIOLOGICAL OR RELATED FACTORS
- Cultural or family health beliefs
- Faulty appraisal
- Impaired thought processes

## Intermittent Constipation Pattern

### DEFINITION
Periodic episodes of hard, dry stools or absence of stools not associated with a pathological state

### DEFINING CHARACTERISTICS
#### Diagnostic Cues
- Reported or observed episodes of hard, dry stools or absence of stools occurring two to three times per month or more frequently
- Straining at stool

#### Supporting Cues
- Painful defecation
- Reported feeling of abdominal or rectal fullness; abdominal distention; back pain
- Reported feeling of pressure in rectum
- Use of laxatives
- Headache
- Appetite impairment
- Abdominal pain, cramps
- Palpable mass
- Nausea

### OUTCOME
#### Bowel Elimination
- Regularity in formation and evacuation of stool

### ETIOLOGICAL OR RELATED FACTORS
- Low-roughage diet
- Low fluid intake
- Absence of routines (time)

## ELIMINATION PATTERN

♦ Decreased activity level
♦ Routine use of enemas, laxatives

## HIGH-RISK POPULATIONS

♦ Hemorrhoids
♦ Antacids
♦ Therapeutic bed rest

## Risk for Constipation (1998)

**DEFINITION**
Presence of risk factors for a decrease in frequency of defecation and difficult or incomplete passage of stool and/or passage of excessively hard, dry stool

**RISK FACTORS**
**Dietary Factors**

- Dehydration, insufficient fiber intake, poor eating habits, change in usual foods and eating patterns
- Decreased motility of gastrointestinal tract
- Inadequate dentition or oral hygiene
- Insufficient fluid intake

**Functional Factors**

- Insufficient physical activity
- Irregular defecation habits (e.g., timeliness)
- Change in usual positioning for defecation
- Loss of privacy
- Abdominal muscle weakness
- Habitual denial or ignoring of urge to defecate
- Recent environmental change influencing habit pattern

**Psychological Factors**

- Depression
- Emotional stress
- Mental confusion
- Aluminum-containing antacids
- Anticholinergics
- Anticonvulsants
- Antidepressants
- Antilipemic agents
- Bismuth salts, calcium carbonate

+ Calcium channel blockers
+ Diuretics, laxative overuse
+ Nonsteroidal anti-inflammatory agents
+ Opiates, sedatives
+ Phenothiazides, sympathomimetics

## Mechanical Factors

+ Obesity, pregnancy, postsurgical obstruction
+ Prostate enlargement
+ Rectal prolapse, rectocele
+ Rectal or anal stricture/fissure/prolapse/abscess
+ Cerebral vascular accident
+ Electrolyte imbalance
+ Hemorrhoids, megacolon (Hirschsprung's disease)

## OUTCOME

## Bowel Elimination

+ Regularity in formation and evacuation of stool

## Diarrhea (1975, 1998)

**DEFINITION**

Passage of loose, unformed stools

**DEFINING CHARACTERISTICS**

**Diagnostic Cues**

- At least three liquid, loose stools per day

**Supporting Cues**

- Hyperactive bowel sounds
- Urgency
- Abdominal pain
- Cramping

**OUTCOME**

**Bowel Elimination**

- Regularity in formation and evacuation of stool

**ETIOLOGICAL OR RELATED FACTORS**

- Laxative abuse
- Tube feedings
- Travel (bacteria, etc. in food and water)
- Alcohol abuse
- High stress or anxiety

**HIGH-RISK POPULATIONS**

- Infectious processes (parasites, toxins)
- Medications
- Inflammation, irritation
- Contaminants
- Radiation
- Malabsorption

## Bowel Incontinence (1975, 1998)

### DEFINITION

Change in bowel habits characterized by involuntary passage of stool

### DEFINING CHARACTERISTICS

#### Diagnostic Cues

+ Involuntary passage of stool

#### Supporting Cues

+ Reports inability to delay defecation
+ Inattention to urge to defecate
+ Inability to recognize urge to defecate
+ Reports inability to feel rectal fullness
+ Recognizes rectal fullness but reports inability to expel formed stool
+ Constant dribbling of soft stool
+ Fecal odor
+ Fecal staining of clothing or bedding
+ Red perianal skin
+ Urgency

### OUTCOME

#### Bowel Continence

+ Control in the passage of stool from the bowel

### ETIOLOGICAL OR RELATED FACTORS

+ Environmental factors (e.g., inaccessible bathroom)
+ Cognitive impairment
+ Abnormally high abdominal or intestinal pressure (from gas)
+ Laxative abuse; dietary habits

*Continues*

### Bowel Incontinence (1975, 1998)—*cont'd*

- Immobility; general decline in muscle tone
  (e.g., abdominal, perineal, bowel sphincter)
- Impaction
- Incomplete emptying of bowel

## HIGH-RISK POPULATIONS

- Chronic diarrhea
- Rectal sphincter abnormality
- Colorectal lesions
- Impaired reservoir (bowel) capacity
- Medications
- Upper/lower motor nerve damage

## Dysfunctional Gastrointestinal Motility* (2008)

### DEFINITION

Increased, decreased, ineffective or lack of peristaltic activity within the gastrointestinal system

### DEFINING CHARACTERISTICS

- ♦ Absence of flatus
- ♦ Abdominal cramping
- ♦ Abdominal distention
- ♦ Abdominal pain
- ♦ Accelerated gastric emptying
- ♦ Bile-colored gastric residual
- ♦ Changes in bowel sounds (e.g., absent, hypoactive, hyperactive)
- ♦ Diarrhea
- ♦ Dry stool
- ♦ Difficulty passing stool
- ♦ Hard stool
- ♦ Increased gastric residual
- ♦ Nausea/vomiting
- ♦ Regurgitation

### OUTCOME

#### Gastrointestinal System

- ♦ Presence of peristaltic activity within gastrointestinal system

### ETIOLOGICAL OR RELATED FACTORS

- ♦ Anxiety
- ♦ Enteral feedings
- ♦ Food intolerance (e.g., gluten, lactose)

*Continues*

*If diagnosed, refer for medical evaluation.

## Dysfunctional Gastrointestinal Motility (2008)—*cont'd*

- Immobility
- Ingestion of contaminates (e.g., food, water)
- Malnutrition
- Pharmaceutical agents (e.g., narcotics/opiates, laxatives, antibiotics, anesthesia)
- Sedentary lifestyle

**HIGH-RISK POPULATIONS**

- Aged
- Prematurity
- Surgery

## Risk for Dysfunctional Gastrointestinal Motility (2008)

### DEFINITION

Risk for increased, decreased, ineffective or lack of peristaltic activity within the gastrointestinal system

### RISK FACTORS

- Anxiety
- Stress
- Unsanitary food preparation
- Change in food
- Change in water
- Food intolerance (e.g., gluten, lactose)
- Gastroesophageal reflux disease
- Sedentary lifestyle
- Immobility
- Infection (e.g., bacterial, parasitic, viral)
- Pharmaceutical agents (e.g., antibiotics, laxatives, narcotics/opiates, proton pump inhibitors)
- Prematurity
- Abdominal surgery
- Aging
- Decreased gastrointestinal circulation
- Diabetes mellitus

### OUTCOME

### Gastrointestinal System

- Presence of peristaltic activity within gastrointestinal system

## Impaired Urinary Elimination (1973)

### DEFINITION

An involuntary loss of urine at somewhat predictable intervals when a specific bladder volume is reached

### DEFINING CHARACTERISTICS

- Incontinence
- Urgency
- Nocturia
- Hesitancy
- Frequency
- Dysuria
- Retention

### ETIOLOGICAL OR RELATED FACTORS

- Urinary tract infection
- Anatomical obstruction
- Multiple causality
- Sensory-motor impairment

### OUTCOME

#### Urinary Elimination

- Predictable discharge of urine

## Functional Incontinence* (1986, 1998)

### DEFINITION

Inability of usually continent person to reach toilet in time to avoid unintentional loss of urine

### DEFINING CHARACTERISTICS

- Reports loss of urine before reaching toilet (accidents)
- Senses need to void but amount of time required to reach toilet exceeds length of time between sensing urge and uncontrolled voiding (loss of urine before reaching toilet)
- May only be incontinent in early morning
- Able to empty bladder completely

### OUTCOME

#### Urinary Continence

- Control and elimination of urine from the bladder

### ETIOLOGICAL OR RELATED FACTORS

- Neuromuscular limitations
- Impaired vision
- Impaired cognition
- Psychological factors
- Environmental factors
- Weakened supporting pelvic structures

*NANDA uses the name Functional Urinary Incontinence.

## Overflow Urinary Incontinence (2007)

### DEFINITION

Involuntary loss of urine associated with over-distention of the bladder

### DEFINING CHARACTERISTICS

- ◆ Bladder distention
- ◆ High postvoid residual volume
- ◆ Nocturia
- ◆ Observed involuntary leakage of small volumes of urine
- ◆ Reports of involuntary leakage of small volumes of urine

### ETIOLOGICAL OR RELATED FACTORS

- ◆ Bladder outlet obstruction
- ◆ Detrusor external sphincter dyssynergia
- ◆ Detrusor hypocontractility
- ◆ Fecal impaction
- ◆ Severe pelvic prolapse
- ◆ Side effects of anticholinergic medications
- ◆ Side effects of calcium channel blockers
- ◆ Side effects of decongestant medications
- ◆ Urethral obstruction

### OUTCOME

**Urinary Continence**

- ◆ Control in the elimination of urine from the bladder

## Reflex Incontinence* (1986, 1998)

### DEFINITION

Involuntary loss of urine at somewhat predictable intervals when a specific bladder volume is reached

### DEFINING CHARACTERISTICS

#### Diagnostic Cues

- Predictable pattern of involuntary loss of urine
- No sensation of urge to void; no sensation of bladder fullness or voiding
- Unable to cognitively inhibit or initiate voiding

#### Supporting Cues

- Sensation of urge to void without voluntary inhibition of bladder contraction
- Sensations associated with full bladder such as sweating, restlessness, and abdominal discomfort
- Incomplete emptying with lesion above sacral micturition center
- Complete emptying with lesion above pontine micturition center

### OUTCOME

#### Urinary Continence

- Control in the elimination of urine from the bladder

### ETIOLOGICAL OR RELATED FACTORS

- Knowledge deficit (bladder management)

### HIGH-RISK POPULATIONS

- Neurological impairment above level of sacral micturition center or pontine micturition center (e.g., myelomeningocele)

*NANDA uses the name Reflex Urinary Incontinence.

## Stress Incontinence* (1986)

### DEFINITION
Involuntary loss of urine of less than 50 mL occurring with increased abdominal pressure

### DEFINING CHARACTERISTICS
#### Diagnostic Cues
+ Reported or observed dribbling with increased abdominal pressure (sneezing, coughing, rising from low chair, laughing)

#### Supporting Cues
+ Report of urinary urgency
+ Urinary frequency (more often than every 2 hours)

### OUTCOME
#### Urinary Continence
+ Control in the elimination of urine from the bladder

### ETIOLOGICAL OR RELATED FACTORS
+ Weak pelvic muscles and structural supports
+ Overdistention between voidings
+ High intra-abdominal pressure (e.g., obesity)

### HIGH-RISK POPULATIONS
+ High intra-abdominal pressure (e.g., gravid uterus)
+ Incompetent bladder outlet
+ Age-related degenerative changes in pelvic muscles/structural supports
+ Weak pelvic muscles and structural supports

*NANDA uses the name Stress Urinary Incontinence.

## Urge Incontinence* (1986)

### DEFINITION

Involuntary passage of urine occurring soon after a strong sense of urgency to void

### DEFINING CHARACTERISTICS

#### Diagnostic Cues

- Inability to reach toilet in time with loss of urine
- Cannot hold or suppress urination urge (urinary urgency)

#### Supporting Cues

- Frequency (voiding more often than every 2 hours)
- Bladder contracture or spasm
- Nocturia (more than two times per night)
- Voiding in small amounts (less than 10 mL) or in large amounts (more than 550 mL)

### OUTCOME

#### Urinary Continence

- Control in the elimination of urine from the bladder

### ETIOLOGICAL OR RELATED FACTORS

- Alcohol, caffeine
- Increased fluid intake
- Increased urine concentration
- Overdistention of bladder

*Continues*

---

*NANDA uses the name Urge Urinary Incontinence.

Urge Incontinence (1986)—*cont'd*

## HIGH-RISK POPULATIONS

- Bladder spasm (irritation of bladder stretch receptors, e.g., bladder infection)
- Decreased bladder capacity (e.g., history of pelvic inflammatory disease, abdominal surgeries, indwelling urinary catheter)

### Risk for Urge Incontinence* (1998)

#### DEFINITION

Risk for involuntary loss of urine associated with a sudden, strong sensation of urgency

#### RISK FACTORS

- Ineffective toileting habits
- Effects of medications (caffeine, alcohol)
- Detrusor hyperreflexia from cystitis
- Detrusor muscle instability with impaired contractility
- Involuntary sphincter relaxation
- Small bladder capacity
- Urethritis
- Tumors, renal calculi
- Central nervous system disorders above pontine, micturition center

#### OUTCOME

#### Urinary Continence

- Control in the elimination of urine from the bladder

*NANDA uses the name Risk for Urge Urinary Incontinence.

## Total Urinary Incontinence (1986)

### DEFINITION
Continuous and unpredictable loss of urine

### DEFINING CHARACTERISTICS
#### Diagnostic Cues
- Constant flow of urine at unpredictable times without distention or uninhibited bladder contractions or spasms
- Lack of perineal or bladder-filling awareness
- Unawareness of incontinence

#### Supporting Cues
- Nocturia
- Unsuccessful incontinence refractory treatments

### OUTCOME
#### Urinary Continence
- Control in the elimination of urine from the bladder

### ETIOLOGICAL OR RELATED FACTORS
- Ineffective incontinence management

### HIGH-RISK POPULATIONS
- Neuropathy, for example, trauma (spinal cord nerves preventing transmission of reflex indicating bladder fullness)
- Neurological dysfunction (triggering micturition at unpredictable times)
- Independent contraction of detrusor reflex (resulting from surgery)

## Urinary Retention* (1986)

### DEFINITION

Incomplete emptying of the bladder

### DEFINING CHARACTERISTICS

#### Diagnostic Cues

♦ Bladder distention
♦ Small, frequent voiding or absence of urine output
♦ Residual urine in bladder (100 mL or more)

#### Supporting Cues

♦ Overflow incontinence
♦ Reports sensation of bladder fullness
♦ Dribbling
♦ Dysuria

### OUTCOME

#### Urinary Continence

♦ Control in the elimination of urine from the bladder

### ETIOLOGICAL OR RELATED FACTORS

♦ High urethral pressure (caused by weak detrusor)
♦ Blockage of urine

### HIGH-RISK POPULATIONS

♦ Inhibition of reflex arc
♦ Strong sphincter

---

*If diagnosed, refer for medical evaluation unless attributable to not taking time to empty bladder when voiding.

**Readiness for Enhanced Urinary Elimination (2002)**

## DEFINITION

Pattern of urinary functions that are sufficient for meeting eliminatory needs and can be strengthened

## DEFINING CHARACTERISTICS

- Expresses willingness to enhance urinary elimination
- Urine is straw colored with no odor
- Specific gravity within normal limits
- Amount of output within normal limits for age/other factors
- Positions self for emptying bladder
- Fluid intake adequate for daily needs

## OUTCOME

### Urinary Elimination

- Collection and discharge of urine at predictable intervals

**NOTES**

## NOTES

# Activity–Exercise Pattern

## Activity Intolerance* (Specify Level) (1982)

### DEFINITION
Abnormal responses to energy-consuming body movements involved in required or desired daily activities

### DEFINING CHARACTERISTICS
#### Diagnostic Cues*

- Report of dyspnea or shortness of breath
- Observation of difficulty breathing with activity
- Report of fatigue (evaluate in context of other cues)
- Heart rate changes (especially with cardiorespiratory problems)
- Muscle weakness, discomfort, pain (especially with neuromusculoskeletal problems) and/or after energy-consuming activity
- Failure of heart rate to return to normal (baseline rate) within approximately 3 minutes after energy-consuming activity

#### Requiring Immediate Attention and Evaluation

- Reports discomfort or chest pain with activity (specify level of activity)
- Arrhythmias with activity (specify level of activity)
- Diastolic pressure increased by 15 mm Hg or more during activity
- Ischemic changes on ECG with activity (specify level of activity)
- Failure of blood pressure to increase with activity
- Dyspnea at rest (unless this is a baseline)

*Although there are a number of studies in nursing, the findings are not consistent on some indicators. Caution should be exercised and the activity stopped if intolerance is suspected.

## ACTIVITY–EXERCISE PATTERN

| | |
|---|---|
| **Level I:** | Walk, regular pace, on level ground indefinitely; one flight or more but more short of breath than normally |
| **Level II:** | Walk one city block 500 feet on level ground; climb one flight slowly without stopping |
| **Level III:** | Walk no more than 50 feet on level ground without stopping; unable to climb one flight of stairs without stopping |
| **Level IV:** | Dyspnea and fatigue at rest |

## OUTCOME

### Activity Tolerance

♦ Physiological response to energy-consuming movements with daily activities; specify level to be attained

## ETIOLOGICAL OR RELATED FACTORS

♦ Generalized weakness
♦ Sedentary lifestyle

## HIGH-RISK POPULATIONS

♦ Imbalance between oxygen supply and demand (e.g., cardiovascular, pulmonary conditions, and changes with aging)
♦ Activity progression (e.g., cardiac and other rehabilitation)
♦ Long-term bed rest or immobility, deconditioned status

### Risk for Activity Intolerance (1982)

**DEFINITION**

Presence of risk factors for abnormal response to energy consuming body movements

**RISK FACTORS**

- Deconditioned status (prolonged bed rest, inactivity)
- Documented respiratory problems
- Documented cardiac problems
- History of previous intolerance to activity
- Documented circulatory problems
- Currently on an activity-progression program
- Desire or need to engage in a higher level of activity
- Inexperience with the activity
- Generalized weakness (chronic disease)

**OUTCOME**

**Activity Tolerance**

- Physiological response to energy-consuming movements with daily activities

## Sedentary Lifestyle  (2004)

### DEFINITION

Reports a habit of life that is characterized by a low physical activity level

### Defining Characteristics

- Chooses a daily routine lacking physical exercise
- Demonstrates physical deconditioning
- Verbalizes preference for activities low in physical activity

### OUTCOME

### Activity Lifestyle

- Thirty minutes per day of physical activity/exercise

### ETIOLOGICAL OR RELATED FACTORS

- Knowledge deficit (health benefits of exercise)
- Lack of training for accomplishment of physical exercise
- Lack of resources (time, money, companionship, facilities)
- Lack of motivation/interest

## ACTIVITY–EXERCISE PATTERN

### Fatigue  (1988, 1998)

## DEFINITION

Overwhelming, sustained sense of exhaustion and decreased capacity for physical and mental work at usual level

## DEFINING CHARACTERISTICS

### Diagnostic Cues

+ Reports unremitting and overwhelming lack of energy
+ Insufficient energy to maintain usual routine (physical activity, required tasks; decreased work performance)

### Supporting Cues

+ Increase in rest requirements; inability to restore energy even after sleep
+ Drowsy, tired, listless
+ Irritable
+ Increase in physical complaints
+ Decreased concentration
+ Compromised libido
+ Disinterest in surroundings
+ Feelings of guilt for not keeping up with responsibilities

## OUTCOME

### Activity Tolerance

+ Absence of fatigue with energy-consuming daily activities

## ETIOLOGICAL AND RELATED FACTORS

### Physiological Factors

+ Sleep deprivation
+ Increased physical exertion
+ Stress

## ACTIVITY–EXERCISE PATTERN

- Anxiety
- Depression
- Boring lifestyle

### Situational Factors

- Negative life events
- Occupation

### Environmental Factors

- Lights, noise during sleep time
- Humidity
- Temperature

### HIGH-RISK POPULATIONS

- Anemia
- Disease states
- Pregnancy

## Deficient Diversional Activity (1980)

### DEFINITION
Decreased engagement in recreational or leisure activities

### DEFINING CHARACTERISTICS
**Diagnostic Cues**
- Expressed wish for something to do, such as read
- Report of boredom or daytime napping

**Supporting Cues**
- States usual hobbies or activities cannot be undertaken (e.g., in hospital)

### OUTCOME
**Leisure Participation**
- Use of relaxing, interesting, and enjoyable activities to promote well-being

### ETIOLOGICAL OR RELATED FACTORS
- Long-term hospitalization apathy
- Environmental lack of diversional activity

### HIGH-RISK POPULATIONS
- Frequent lengthy treatments
- Long-term illness
- High job and/or family demands

> ## Impaired Physical Mobility (Specify Level) (1973, 1998)

### DEFINITION

Limitation of independent, purposeful body movement in the environment

### DEFINING CHARACTERISTICS

#### Diagnostic Cues

- Inability to move within the physical environment
- Postural instability during performance of routine activities
- Decreased muscle control, strength or mass

#### Supporting Cues

- Gait changes, for example, decreased walk speed, difficulty initiating gait, small steps, shuffles feet, exaggerated lateral postural sway
- Reluctance to initiate movement, for example, fear, insufficient self-efficacy
- Engages in substitutions for movement, for example, fixation on activity, increased attention to other's activity, controlling behavior, focus on preillness or predisability activity

#### Functional Level Classification

| | |
|---|---|
| **Level I:** | Requires use of equipment or device |
| **Level II:** | Requires help from another person for assistance, supervision, or teaching |
| **Level III:** | Requires help from another person and equipment or device |
| **Level IV:** | Dependent; does not participate in activity |

*Continues*

## Impaired Physical Mobility (Specify Level) (1973, 1998)—cont'd

## OUTCOME

### Mobility

- ♦ Ability to move purposefully in own environment independently with or without assistive device (specify Level to be attained)

## ETIOLOGICAL OR RELATED FACTORS

- ♦ Activity intolerance (e.g., movement-induced shortness of breath; limited cardiovascular endurance)
- ♦ Joint stiffness or contractures (limited range of motion)
- ♦ Pain, discomfort
- ♦ Musculoskeletal impairment (e.g., loss of integrity of bone structures)
- ♦ Neuromuscular impairment (e.g., limited ability to perform fine/gross motor skills, uncoordinated or jerky movements, movement-induced tremor)
- ♦ Cognitive–sensory-perceptual impairment (e.g., decreased reaction time)
- ♦ Depressive mood state or anxiety
- ♦ Sedentary lifestyle, disuse, deconditioning
- ♦ Body mass index above 75th age-appropriate percentile
- ♦ Prescribed movement restriction, for example, physical or chemical restraints, bed rest prescription, use of mechanical equipment that restricts movement, therapeutic immobilization

## Impaired Bed Mobility (Specify Level) (1998)

### DEFINITION

Limitation of independent movement from one bed position to another

### DEFINING CHARACTERISTICS

#### Diagnostic Cues

One or more of the following:

- ♦ Impaired ability to turn side to side
- ♦ Impaired ability to move from supine to sitting or sitting to supine
- ♦ Impaired ability to "scoot" or reposition self in bed
- ♦ Impaired ability to move from supine to prone or prone to supine
- ♦ Impaired ability to move from supine to long sitting or long sitting to supine

#### Functional Level Classification

| | |
|---|---|
| **Level I:** | Requires use of equipment or device |
| **Level II:** | Requires help from another person(s) for assistance, supervision, teaching |
| **Level III:** | Requires help from another person(s) and equipment or device |
| **Level IV:** | Dependent; does not participate in movement |

### OUTCOME

#### Body Positioning: Self-Initiated

- ♦ Ability to change own body position independently with or without assistive device (specify level to be attained)

*Continues*

## Impaired Bed Mobility (Specify Level) (1998)—*cont'd*

### ETIOLOGICAL OR RELATED FACTORS

- None

### HIGH-RISK POPULATIONS

- Paralysis
- Weakness
- Coma
- Marked weakness
- Marked obesity

## Impaired Transfer Ability (Specify Level) (1998)

### DEFINITION

Limitation of independent body movement between two nearby surfaces

### DEFINING CHARACTERISTICS

#### Diagnostic Cues

One or more of the following:

- Impaired ability to transfer from bed to chair and chair to bed
- Impaired ability to transfer on or off a toilet or commode
- Impaired ability to transfer in and out of tub or shower
- Impaired ability to transfer between uneven levels
- Impaired ability to transfer from chair to car or car to chair
- Impaired ability to transfer from chair to floor or floor to chair
- Impaired ability to transfer from standing to floor or floor to standing

#### Functional Level Classification

| | |
|---|---|
| **Level I:** | Requires use of equipment or device |
| **Level II:** | Requires help from another person(s) for assistance, supervision, teaching |
| **Level III:** | Requires help from another person(s) and equipment or device |
| **Level IV:** | Dependent; does not participate in movement |

*Continues*

## Impaired Transfer Ability (Specify Level) (1998)—*cont'd*

### OUTCOME

#### Transfer Performance

- ◆ Ability to change body location independently with or without assistive device (specify level to be attained)

### ETIOLOGICAL OR RELATED FACTORS

- ◆ None

### HIGH-RISK POPULATIONS

- ◆ Paralysis
- ◆ Peripheral sensory loss
- ◆ Marked weakness
- ◆ Marked obesity

## Impaired Wheelchair Mobility  (1998)

### DEFINITION

Limitation of independent operation of wheelchair within the environment

### DEFINING CHARACTERISTICS

#### Diagnostic Cues

One or more of the following:

- Impaired ability to operate manual or power wheelchair on even or uneven surface
- Impaired ability to operate manual or power wheelchair on an incline or decline
- Impaired ability to operate wheelchair on curbs

### OUTCOME

#### Ambulation: Wheelchair

- Ability to move from place to place using a wheelchair (specify level to be attained)

### ETIOLOGICAL OR RELATED FACTORS

- None

### HIGH-RISK POPULATIONS

- Sensory or neuromuscular loss (e.g., spinal cord injury, muscular dystrophy, cerebral vascular accident)
- Marked weakness
- Severe arthritis

## Impaired Walking (Specify Level) (1998)

### DEFINITION

Limitation of independent movement within the environment on foot (or with a device, e.g., cane, crutches, walker)

### DEFINING CHARACTERISTICS

#### Diagnostic Cues

One or more of the following:

- ♦ Impaired ability to climb stairs
- ♦ Impaired ability to walk required distances
- ♦ Impaired ability to walk on an incline or decline
- ♦ Impaired ability to walk on uneven surfaces
- ♦ Impaired ability to navigate curbs

#### Functional Level Classification

| | |
|---|---|
| **Level I:** | Requires use of equipment or device (cane, crutches, walker) |
| **Level II:** | Requires help from another person(s) for assistance, supervision, teaching |
| **Level III:** | Requires help from another person(s) and equipment or device |
| **Level IV:** | Dependent; does not participate in movement |

### OUTCOME

#### Mobility

- ♦ Ability to move purposefully in own environment independently with or without assistive device (specify level to be attained)

### ETIOLOGICAL OR RELATED FACTORS

- ♦ Cognitive impairment
- ♦ Impaired balance

## ACTIVITY–EXERCISE PATTERN

- Deconditioning
- Environmental constraints (e.g., stairs, inclines, uneven surfaces, unsafe obstacles, restraints, distances, lack of assistive devices or person)
- Fear (falling)
- Insufficient muscle strength
- Limited endurance
- Contractures
- Muscular skeletal or neuromuscular impairment
- Obesity
- Pain
- Deficient knowledge

## HIGH-RISK POPULATIONS

- Sensory-motor loss
- Severe arthritis
- Severe weakness
- Limb amputation

### Wandering (2000)

#### DEFINITION

Meandering, aimless, or repetitive locomotion that exposes the individual to harm; frequently incongruent with boundaries, limits, or obstacles; may be sporadic or continual

#### DEFINING CHARACTERISTICS

#### Diagnostic Cues

One or more of the following:

- Frequent or continuous movement from place to place, often revisiting the same destinations
- Persistent locomotion in search of "missing" or unattainable people
- Haphazard locomotion
- Locomotion into unauthorized or private spaces
- Locomotion resulting in unintended leaving of premises
- Long periods of locomotion without an apparent destination
- Locomotion that cannot be easily dissuaded or redirected
- Following behind or shadowing a caregiver's locomotion
- Hyperactivity
- Scanning, seeking, or searching behaviors
- Periods of locomotion interspersed with periods of nonlocomotion (e.g., sitting, standing, sleeping)
- Multiple episodes of getting lost

## Supporting Cues

- Trespassing
- Fretful locomotion or pacing
- Inability to locate significant landmarks in a familiar setting

## OUTCOME

### Safe Home Environment

- Physical arrangements minimize environmental factors that might cause physical harm or injury in the house/community

## ETIOLOGICAL OR RELATED FACTORS

- Cognitive impairment specifically memory and recall deficits, disorientation, poor visuoconstructive (or visuospatial) ability, language defects (primarily expressive)
- Cortical atrophy
- Premorbid behavior (e.g., outgoing, sociable personality; premorbid dementia)
- Separation from familiar people and places
- Sedation
- Frustration, anxiety, boredom, depression (agitation)
- Overstimulating/understimulating social or physical environment
- Physiological state or need (e.g., hunger/thirst, pain, urination, constipation)
- Time of day

## Risk for Disuse Syndrome* (1988)

### DEFINITION

Presence of risk factors for deterioration of body systems as the result of prescribed or unavoidable musculoskeletal inactivity

### RISK FACTORS

- Paralysis
- Mechanical immobilization (e.g., lower-body cast, leg traction, vascular lines)
- Prescribed immobilization
- Severe pain
- Altered level of consciousness
- Severe depression

### OUTCOME

### Immobility Consequences: Physiological/ Psychocognitive

- Normal physiological/psychocognitive functioning

*Complications of immobility can include pressure ulcer, constipation, stasis of pulmonary secretions, thrombosis, urinary tract infection and/or retention, decreased strength or endurance, orthostatic hypotension, decreased range of joint motion, disorientation, body image disturbance, and powerlessness.

## Risk for Joint Contractures

### DEFINITION

Presence of risk factors for shortening of tendons at movable joints (back, head, upper and lower extremities)

### RISK FACTORS

- Loss of voluntary postural muscle control
- Prolonged joint flexion in sitting or recumbent position
- Spasticity
- Report of pain or discomfort on movement
- Imposed restrictions of joint movement (e.g., casts, traction)
- Assumption of abnormal posture resulting from psychosocial factors or cognitive deficit

### OUTCOME

**Joint Motion**

- Functional range of joint motion

## Self Neglect  (2008)

### DEFINITION

A constellation of culturally framed behaviors involving one
or more self-care activities in which there is a failure to maintain a socially accepted standard of health and well-being
(Gibbons, Lauder, & Ludwick, 2006)

### DEFINING CHARACTERISTICS

+ Inadequate personal hygiene
+ Inadequate environmental hygiene
+ Nonadherence to health activities

### OUTCOME

### Self-Care: Hygiene

+ Maintains own personal cleanliness and appearance
  with or without assistive device(s)

### ETIOLOGICAL OR RELATED FACTORS

+ Functional impairment
+ Lifestyle/choice
+ Capgras syndrome
+ Cognitive impairment (e.g., dementia)
+ Depression
+ Learning disability
+ Fear (institutionalization)
+ Maintaining control
+ Malingering
+ Substance abuse
+ Major life stressor

## ACTIVITY–EXERCISE PATTERN

### HIGH-RISK POPULATIONS

- Frontal lobe dysfunction and executive processing ability
- Schizotypal personality disorders
- Paranoid personality disorders
- Obsessive-compulsive disorder
- Depression

## Total Self-Care Deficit (Specify Level)

### DEFINITION

Inability to complete feeding, bathing, toileting, dressing, and grooming of self

### DEFINING CHARACTERISTICS

#### Diagnostic Cues

Observation or valid report of inability to eat, bathe, toilet, dress, and groom self independently (see defining characteristics for each deficit on pp. 199–206)

#### Functional Level Classification

| | |
|---|---|
| **Level I:** | Requires use of equipment or devices |
| **Level II:** | Requires help from another person(s) for assistance, supervision, teaching |
| **Level III:** | Requires help from another person(s) and equipment or device |
| **Level IV:** | Dependent; does not participate in self-care |

### OUTCOME

#### Self-Care

+ Completes feeding, bathing, toileting, dressing, and grooming of self (specify level to be attained)

### ETIOLOGICAL OR RELATED FACTORS

+ Decreased activity tolerance, strength, and/or endurance
+ Pain or discomfort
+ Uncompensated perceptual-cognitive impairment (specify)

## ACTIVITY–EXERCISE PATTERN

- Uncompensated neuromuscular impairment (specify)
- Uncompensated musculoskeletal impairment (specify)
- Severe anxiety
- Depression
- Environmental barriers

## Bathing–Hygiene Self-Care Deficit (Specify Level) (1980, 1998)

### DEFINITION

Impaired ability to perform or complete bathing and hygiene activities

### DEFINING CHARACTERISTICS

#### Diagnostic Cues

♦ Impaired ability to wash body or body parts

and one or more of the following:

- ♦ Impaired ability to obtain water
- ♦ Impaired ability to get to water source (tub, shower, sink)
- ♦ Impaired ability to regulate water temperature or flow

#### Functional Level Classification

| | |
|---|---|
| Level I: | Requires use of equipment or devices |
| Level II: | Requires help from another person(s) for assistance, supervision, teaching |
| Level III: | Requires help from another person(s) and equipment or device |
| Level IV: | Dependent; does not participate in self-care bathing or hygiene |

### OUTCOME

#### Self-Care: Bathing

♦ Cleanses own body independently with or without assistive device (specify level to be attained)

## ACTIVITY–EXERCISE PATTERN

### Self-Care: Hygiene

- Maintains own personal cleanliness and appearance independently with or without assistive device (specify level to be attained)

### ETIOLOGICAL OR RELATED FACTORS

- Decreased activity tolerance, strength, and/or endurance
- Pain or discomfort
- Uncompensated perceptual-cognitive impairment (specify)
- Uncompensated neuromuscular impairment (specify)
- Uncompensated musculoskeletal impairment (specify)
- Severe anxiety
- Depression
- Environmental barriers

# ACTIVITY–EXERCISE PATTERN

## Dressing–Grooming Self-Care Deficit (Specify Level) (1980, 1998)

### DEFINITION

Impaired ability to perform or complete dressing and grooming activities

### DEFINING CHARACTERISTICS

#### Diagnostic Cues

Inability to

- Choose clothing
- Pick up clothing
- Put on and take off necessary items of clothing on upper body
- Put on and take off necessary items of clothing on lower body (put on socks and shoes)
- Fasten clothing and use zippers

#### Supporting Cues

- Obtain or replace items of clothing (situation dependent)
- Maintain appearance at a satisfactory level

#### Functional Level Classification

| | |
|---|---|
| Level I: | Requires use of equipment or device |
| Level II: | Requires help from another person for assistance, supervision, or teaching |
| Level III: | Requires help from another person and equipment or device |
| Level IV: | Dependent; does not participate in self-dressing or grooming |

# ACTIVITY–EXERCISE PATTERN

## OUTCOME

### Self-Care: Dressing

- Dresses self independently with or without assistive device (specify level to be attained)

## ETIOLOGICAL OR RELATED FACTORS

- Decreased activity tolerance, strength, and or endurance (weakness or tiredness)
- Pain, discomfort
- Uncompensated perceptual or cognitive impairment
- Uncompensated neuromuscular impairment
- Uncompensated musculoskeletal impairment
- Severe anxiety
- Environmental barriers
- Situational depression
- Decreased motivation or lack of motivation

## Feeding Self-Care Deficit (Specify Level)  (1980, 1998)

### DEFINITION

Impaired ability to perform or complete feeding activities

### DEFINING CHARACTERISTICS

#### Diagnostic Cues

♦ Inability to bring food from receptacle to the mouth

#### Supporting Cues

♦ Inability to prepare food for ingestion
♦ Inability to open containers
♦ Inability to get food onto utensil and handle utensils
♦ Inability to pick up cup or glass
♦ Inability to complete a meal
♦ Inability to ingest food in a socially acceptable manner
♦ Inability to ingest food safely
♦ Inability to ingest sufficient food

#### Functional Level Classification

| | |
|---|---|
| **Level I:** | Requires use of equipment or device |
| **Level II:** | Requires help from another person for assistance, supervision, or teaching |
| **Level III:** | Requires help from another person and equipment or device |
| **Level IV:** | Dependent; does not participate in self-feeding |

### OUTCOME

#### Self-Care: Eating

♦ Prepares and ingests food and fluid independently with or without assistive device (specify level to be attained)

210

## ACTIVITY–EXERCISE PATTERN

### ETIOLOGICAL OR RELATED FACTORS

- ◆ Decreased activity tolerance, strength, and/or endurance (weakness or tiredness)
- ◆ Pain, discomfort
- ◆ Uncompensated perceptual or cognitive impairment
- ◆ Uncompensated neuromuscular impairment
- ◆ Uncompensated musculoskeletal impairment
- ◆ Severe anxiety
- ◆ Environmental barriers
- ◆ Situational depression
- ◆ Decreased motivation or lack of motivation

## Toileting Self-Care Deficit (Specify Level) (1980, 1998)

### DEFINITION

Impaired ability to perform or complete toileting activities

### DEFINING CHARACTERISTICS

#### Diagnostic Cues

- Unable to get to toilet or commode
- Unable to carry out proper toilet hygiene
- Unable to manipulate clothing for toileting
- Unable to rise from toilet or commode

#### Supporting Cues

- Impaired ability to sit on toilet or commode
- Unable to flush toilet or empty commode

#### Functional Level Classification

| | |
|---|---|
| **Level I:** | Requires use of equipment or devices |
| **Level II:** | Requires help from another person(s): assistance, supervision, teaching |
| **Level III:** | Requires help from another person(s) and equipment or device |
| **Level IV:** | Dependent; does not participate in self-toileting |

### OUTCOME

#### Self-Care: Toileting

- Toilets self independently with or without assistive device (specify level to be attained)

### ETIOLOGICAL OR RELATED FACTORS

- Impaired transfer or mobility
- Pain or discomfort

## ACTIVITY–EXERCISE PATTERN

- Decreased activity tolerance, strength, and/or endurance (weakness or tiredness)
- Pain, discomfort
- Uncompensated perceptual or cognitive impairment
- Uncompensated neuromuscular impairment
- Uncompensated musculoskeletal impairment
- Severe anxiety
- Environmental barriers
- Situational depression
- Decreased, or lack, of motivation

## Developmental Delay: Self-Care Skills (Specify Level)

### DEFINITION

Demonstrates deviations from age-group norms for self-care skills

### DEFINING CHARACTERISTICS

#### Diagnostic Cues

- Delay or difficulty in performing self-care skills typical of age-group or developmental level (eating, bathing and hygiene, toileting, dressing, and grooming)

#### Supporting Cues

- Flat affect
- Listlessness
- Decreased responses

#### Functional Level Classification

| | |
|---|---|
| **Level I:** | Requires use of equipment or devices |
| **Level II:** | Requires help from another person(s): assistance, supervision, teaching |
| **Level III:** | Requires help from another person(s) and equipment or device |
| **Level IV:** | Dependent; does not participate in self-toileting |

### OUTCOME

#### Self-Care

- Performs basic personal care activities consistent with age-group norms (specify level to be attained)

### ETIOLOGICAL OR RELATED FACTORS

- Low-stimulation environment (social, physical)
- Environmental and stimulation deficiencies

## ACTIVITY–EXERCISE PATTERN

- Inadequate care taking
- Indifference
- Inconsistent responsiveness
- Multiple caretakers
- Separation (from significant others)
- Physical disability effects
- Prescribed dependence

## ACTIVITY–EXERCISE PATTERN

### Readiness for Enhanced Self-Care (2007)

**DEFINITION**

Pattern of performing activities for oneself that helps to meet health-related goals and can be strengthened

**DEFINING CHARACTERISTICS**

- Expresses desire to enhance independence in maintaining life
- Expresses desire to enhance independence in maintaining health
- Expresses desire to enhance independence in maintaining personal development
- Expresses desire to enhance knowledge of strategies for self-care
- Expresses desire to enhance responsibility for self-care
- Expresses desire to enhance self-care

**OUTCOME**

- Completes self-care independently

# ACTIVITY–EXERCISE PATTERN

## Delayed Surgical Recovery (1998)

### DEFINITION

Extension of the number of postoperative days required for individuals to initiate and perform activities that maintain life, health, and well-being

### DEFINING CHARACTERISTICS

- Difficulty in moving about
- Requires help to complete self-care
- Fatigue
- Report of pain or discomfort
- Postpones resumption of work or play (child)
- Reports perception that more time is needed to recover
- Evidence of interrupted healing of surgical area (e.g., red, indurated, draining, immobile)

### OUTCOME

#### Postprocedure: Recovery Status

- Returns to baseline function following a procedure(s) requiring anesthesia or sedation

### ETIOLOGICAL OR RELATED FACTORS

- To be developed (may be the probable cause of other problems—an etiological factor)

### Delayed Growth and Development* (1986)

**DEFINITION**

Deviations in norms from his or her age group

**DEFINING CHARACTERISTICS**

- Delay or difficulty in performing skills (motor, social, or expressive) typical of age group
- Altered physical growth
- Inability to perform self-care or self-control activities appropriate for age

**OUTCOME**

**Growth**

- Meets milestones of physical, cognitive, and psychosocial progression

**ETIOLOGICAL OR RELATED FACTORS**

- Inadequate care taking
- Indifference
- Inconsistent responsiveness
- Multiple caretakers
- Separation (from significant others)
- Environmental and stimulation deficiencies
- Physical disability effects
- Prescribed dependence

*See Developmental Delay: Social Skills, Language Skills, Communication Skills.

**Risk for Delayed Development\*  (1998)**

## DEFINITION

Risk for delay of 25% or more in one or more of the areas of social or self-regulatory behavior, or cognitive, language, gross, or fine motor skills

## RISK FACTORS

### Prenatal Factors

- Maternal age younger than 15 or older than 35 years
- Substance abuse
- Genetic or endocrine disorders
- Maternal inadequate nutrition
- Late, poor, or lack of prenatal care
- Illiteracy, poverty

### Physiological Factors

- Malnutrition, failure to thrive
- Seizures
- Positive drug screening test
- Brain damage (e.g., hemorrhage in postnatal period, shaken baby, abuse, accident)
- Vision or hearing impairment or frequent otitis media
- Technology dependent
- Lead poisoning
- Prematurity
- Chemotherapy, radiation therapy

### Psychosocial Factors

- Deprivation
- Violence

*Continues*

*See Developmental Delay: Social Skills, Language Skills, Communication Skills.

### Risk for Delayed Development (1998)—*cont'd*

- ◆ Behavior disorders
- ◆ Natural disaster
- ◆ Caregiver mental illness, retardation, severe learning disability
- ◆ Foster or adopted child

## OUTCOME

### Neglect Recovery

- ◆ Development consistent with age norms

### Risk for Disproportionate Growth (1998)

#### DEFINITION

Risk for growth above the 97th percentile or below the 3rd percentile for age, crossing two percentile channels (disproportionate growth)

#### RISK FACTORS

#### Prenatal Factors

- ♦ Congenital or genetic disorders
- ♦ Maternal nutrition
- ♦ Multiple gestation
- ♦ Teratogen exposure
- ♦ Maternal substance use or abuse

#### Physiological Factors

- ♦ Malnutrition
- ♦ Maladaptive feeding behaviors
- ♦ Anorexia
- ♦ Insatiable appetite
- ♦ Infection
- ♦ Chronic illness
- ♦ Lead poisoning
- ♦ Prematurity

#### Psychosocial Factors

- ♦ Deprivation
- ♦ Violence
- ♦ Natural disasters
- ♦ Caregiver abuse
- ♦ Caregiver mental illness, retardation, severe learning disability

*Continues*

**Risk for Disproportionate Growth (1998)—*cont'd***

**OUTCOME**

**Growth**

+ Normal increase in bone size and body weight during growth years

## Impaired Home Maintenance (1980)

### DEFINITION

Inability to independently maintain a safe, growth-promoting immediate environment (specify mild, moderate, severe, potential, chronic)

### DEFINING CHARACTERISTICS

#### Diagnostic Cues

- Household members express difficulty in maintaining their home in a comfortable fashion
- Household members request assistance with home maintenance and one or more of the following:
  - Disorderly surroundings; repeated hygienic disorders, infestations, or infections
  - Offensive odors; accumulation of dirt, food wastes, or hygienic wastes
  - Inappropriate household temperature; unwashed or unavailable cooking equipment, clothes, or linen
  - Overtaxed family members (e.g., exhausted, anxious)
  - Lack of necessary equipment or aids
  - Presence of vermin or rodents
  - Household members describe outstanding debts or financial crises

### OUTCOME

#### Self-Care: Instrumental Activities of Daily Living

- Performs activities needed to function in the home or community independently with or without assistive device

*Continues*

## Impaired Home Maintenance (1980)—*cont'd*

### ETIOLOGICAL OR RELATED FACTORS

- Individual or family member illness or injury
- Support system deficit
- Insufficient family organization or planning
- Insufficient finances, outstanding debts; financial crises
- Unfamiliarity with neighborhood resources
- Impaired cognitive or emotional functioning
- Knowledge deficit (specify area)
- Lack of role modeling

### HIGH-RISK POPULATIONS

- Chronic debilitating illness with fatigue
- History of lack of role models for home management

## Dysfunctional Ventilatory Weaning Response (1992)

### DEFINITION

Inability to adjust to lowered levels of mechanical ventilator support, which interrupts and prolongs the weaning process (mild, moderate, severe)

### DEFINING CHARACTERISTICS

#### Diagnostic Cues

*Mild*

Responds to lowered levels of mechanical ventilator support with

- Restlessness
- Slight increase in respiratory rate from baseline and may report or observe one or more of the following:
  - Expression of increased need for oxygen, breathing discomfort, fatigue, warmth
  - Queries about possible machine malfunction
  - Increased concentration on breathing

*Moderate*

Responds to lowered levels of mechanical ventilator support with

- Slight increase from baseline blood pressure (< 20 mm Hg)
- Slight increase from baseline heart rate (< 20 beats/min)
- Baseline increase in respiratory rate (< 5 breaths/min) and one or more of the following:
  - Hypervigilance to activities
  - Inability to respond to coaching
  - Inability to cooperate
  - Apprehension

*Continues*

**Dysfunctional Ventilatory Weaning Response
(1992)—*cont'd***

- Diaphoresis
- Eye widening ("wide-eyed look")
- Decreased air entry on auscultation
- Color changes (pale, slight cyanosis)
- Slight respiratory accessory muscle use

### *Severe*

Responds to lowered levels of mechanical ventilator
support with

- Agitation
- Deterioration in arterial blood gases from current
  baseline
- Increase from baseline blood pressure 20 mm Hg
- Increase from baseline heart rate 20 beats/minute
- Respiratory rate increases significantly from baseline

and one or more of the following:

- Profuse diaphoresis
- Full respiratory accessory muscle use
- Shallow, gasping breaths
- Paradoxical abdominal breathing
- Discoordinated breathing with the ventilator
- Decreased level of consciousness
- Adventitious breath sounds, audible airway secretions
- Cyanosis

### Supporting Cues

- History of ventilator dependence 1 week
- History of multiple unsuccessful weaning attempts

# ACTIVITY–EXERCISE PATTERN

## OUTCOME

### Mechanical Ventilation Weaning Response: Adult

- Respiratory and psychological adjustment to progressive removal of mechanical ventilation

## ETIOLOGICAL OR RELATED FACTORS

### Physiological Factors

- Ineffective airway clearance
- Disturbed sleep pattern
- Inadequate nutrition
- Uncontrolled pain or discomfort

### Psychological Factors

- Knowledge deficit (weaning process, patient role)
- Perceived inability to wean
- Decreased motivation
- Decreased self-esteem
- Anxiety: moderate, severe
- Fear
- Hopelessness
- Powerlessness
- Insufficient trust in the nurse

### Situational Factors

- Uncontrolled episodic energy demands or problems
- Inappropriate pacing of diminished ventilator support
- Inadequate social support
- Adverse environment (e.g., noisy, active environment; negative events in the room; low nurse/patient ratio; extended nurse absence from bedside; unfamiliar nursing staff)

## HIGH-RISK POPULATIONS

- Prolonged ventilator dependency
- Severe chronic pulmonary disease

## Impaired Spontaneous Ventilation* (1992)

### DEFINITION

Decreased energy or reserves resulting in an individual's inability to maintain breathing adequate to support life

### DEFINING CHARACTERISTICS

- Dyspnea
- Increased metabolic rate
- Increased restlessness
- Apprehension
- Increased use of accessory muscles
- Decreased tidal volume
- Increased heart rate
- Decreased $pO_2$
- Increased $pCO_2$
- Decreased $SaO_2$

### OUTCOME

#### Respiratory Status: Gas Exchange

- Alveolar exchange of carbon dioxide and oxygen maintains arterial blood gas concentration

### ETIOLOGICAL OR RELATED FACTORS

- Metabolic factors (specify)
- Respiratory muscle fatigue

*If diagnosed, refer for immediate medical evaluation.

## Ineffective Airway Clearance (1980, 1996, 1998)

### DEFINITION

Inability to effectively clear secretions or obstruction from respiratory tract

### DEFINING CHARACTERISTICS

### Diagnostic Cues

- ♦ Adventitious breath sounds (specify location): crackles (rales), rhonchi, wheezes
- ♦ Unable to clear airways; cough ineffective or absent

Progressing to

- ♦ Reports shortness of breath or difficulty breathing
- ♦ Requires frequent suctioning
- ♦ Respiratory rate increase (tachypnea) or depth changes
- ♦ Decreased breath sounds
- ♦ Hypoxemia

### Supporting Cues

- ♦ Dyspnea at rest or on exertion
- ♦ Hypercapnia
- ♦ Cyanosis

### OUTCOME

### Respiratory Status: Airway Patency

- ♦ Open, clear tracheobronchial passages for air exchange

*Continues*

**Ineffective Airway Clearance  (1980, 1996, 1998)—*cont'd***

## ETIOLOGICAL OR RELATED FACTORS

- ♦ Ineffective cough
- ♦ Excess thick secretions
- ♦ Decreased energy or fatigue
- ♦ Pain (specify area)
- ♦ Presence of artificial airway

## HIGH-RISK POPULATIONS

- ♦ Airway obstruction
- ♦ Tracheobronchial infection
- ♦ Trauma
- ♦ Perceptual or cognitive impairment

## Ineffective Breathing Pattern (1980, 1996, 1998)

### DEFINITION

Inspiration and/or expiration that does not provide adequate ventilation

### DEFINING CHARACTERISTICS

#### Diagnostic Cues

- Reports shortness of breath/difficulty breathing
- Dyspnea at rest or on exertion
- Respiratory rate and/or depth changes
- Use of accessory muscles to breathe
- Respiratory rate/min
  - Infants: < 25 or > 60
  - Ages 1–4: < 20 or > 30
  - Ages 5–14: < 14 or > 25
  - Adults > 14 yrs: ≤ 11 or > 24
- Depth of breathing
  - Adult tidal volume: 500 ml at rest
  - Infant tidal volume: 6–8 ml/kg
- Timing ratio
- Decreased vital capacity
- Nasal flaring
- Reports feeling anxious or apprehensive
- Decreased inspiratory/expiratory pressure
- Decreased minute ventilation

#### Supporting Cues

- Pursed-lip breathing
- Reduced motion of chest, prolonged expiratory phase
- Cyanosis
- Orthopnea

*Continues*

## Ineffective Breathing Pattern (1980, 1996, 1998)—*cont'd*

- Nasal flaring
- Abnormal arterial blood gases
- Fremitus
- Increased anteroposterior chest diameter
- Assumption of three-point position

## OUTCOME

### Respiratory Status: Gas Exchange/Ventilation

- Alveolar exchange of carbon dioxide and oxygen maintains arterial blood gas concentrations
- Movement of air in and out of the lungs

## ETIOLOGICAL OR RELATED FACTORS

- Anxiety
- Decreased energy or fatigue
- Pain
- Knowledge deficit (compensatory breathing patterns)
- Bone deformity
- Obesity
- Spinal cord injury
- Body position
- Respiratory muscle fatigue

## HIGH-RISK POPULATIONS

- Neuromusculoskeletal impairment (e.g., spinal cord injury, bony deformity, neurological immaturity)
- Perceptual or cognitive impairment
- Respiratory muscle fatigue
- Chest wall deformity
- Hyperventilation
- Hypoventilation syndrome

## ACTIVITY–EXERCISE PATTERN

### Impaired Gas Exchange* (1980, 1996, 1998)

#### DEFINITION

Excess or deficit in oxygenation and/or carbon dioxide elimination at the alveolar–capillary level

#### DEFINING CHARACTERISTICS

- Reports shortness of breath or difficulty breathing
- Abnormal respiratory rate/rhythm/depth (specify)
- Dyspnea
- Hypoxemia
- Hypercapnia
- Abnormal blood gases, abnormal arterial pH
- Abnormal skin color (pale, dusky, cyanosis)
- Diaphoresis
- Visual disturbances
- Tachycardia
- Restlessness, anxiety
- Confusion, somnolence, irritability
- Headache when awakening

#### OUTCOME

#### Respiratory Status: Gas Exchange

- Alveolar exchange of carbon dioxide and oxygen maintains arterial blood gas concentrations

#### ETIOLOGICAL OR RELATED FACTORS

- Ventilation–perfusion imbalance
- Alveolar–capillary changes

*If diagnosed, refer for medical evaluation.

## Decreased Cardiac Output* (1975, 1996, 2000)

### DEFINITION

Inadequate blood pumped by the heart to meet the metabolic demands of the body

### DEFINING CHARACTERISTICS

#### Altered Heart Rate/Rhythm

- Arrhythmias (tachycardia, bradycardia)
- Palpitations
- EKG changes

#### Altered Preload

- Jugular vein distention
- Fatigue
- Edema
- Murmurs
- Increased/decreased central venous pressure (CVP)
- Increased/decreased pulmonary artery wedge pressure (PAWP)
- Weight gain

#### Altered Afterload

- Cold/clammy skin
- Shortness of breath/dyspnea
- Oliguria
- Prolonged capillary refill
- Decreased peripheral pulses
- Variations in blood pressure readings
- Increased/decreased systemic vascular resistance (SVR)

*If diagnosed, refer for medical evaluation.

- Increased/decreased pulmonary vascular resistance (PVR)
- Skin color changes (pallor)

## Altered Contractility

- Crackles
- Cough
- Orthopnea/paroxysmal nocturnal dyspnea
- Cardiac output < 4 L/min
- Cardiac index < 2.5 L/min
- Decreased ejection fraction
- Stroke Volume Index (SVI)
- Left Ventricular Stroke Work Index (LVSWI)
- S3 or S4 sounds

## Behavioral/Emotional

- Restlessness
- Anxiety

## OUTCOME

### Cardiac Pump Effectiveness

- Adequate blood volume ejected from the left ventricle to support systemic perfusion pressure

## ETIOLOGICAL OR RELATED FACTORS

- (Factors listed by NANDA are same as defining characteristics)

# ACTIVITY–EXERCISE PATTERN

## Risk for Shock (2008)

### DEFINITION

At risk for an inadequate blood flow to the body's tissues, which may lead to a life-threatening cellular dysfunction

### RISK FACTORS

- Hypotension
- Hypovolemia
- Hypoxemia
- Hypoxia
- Infection
- Sepsis
- Systemic inflammatory response syndrome

### OUTCOME

**Circulation**

- Adequate blood flow to body tissues

## Ineffective Peripheral Tissue Perfusion (2008)

### DEFINITION

Decrease in blood circulation to the periphery that may compromise health

### DEFINING CHARACTERISTICS

- Absent pulses
- Altered motor function
- Altered skin characteristics (color, elasticity, hair, moisture, nails, sensation, temperature)
- Blood pressure changes in extremities
- Claudication
- Color does not return to leg on lowering it
- Delayed peripheral wound healing
- Diminished pulses
- Edema
- Extremity pain
- Paraesthesia
- Skin color pale on elevation

### OUTCOME

#### Circulation

- Skin temperature and color within normal limits

### ETIOLOGICAL OR RELATED FACTORS

- Deficient knowledge of aggravating factors (e.g., smoking, sedentary lifestyle, trauma, obesity, salt intake, immobility)
- Deficient knowledge (disease process, e.g., diabetes, hyperlipidemia)

## Risk for Decreased Cardiac Tissue Perfusion (2008)

### DEFINITION

Risk for a decrease in cardiac (coronary) circulation

### RISK FACTORS

- Birth control pills
- Drug abuse
- Elevated C-reactive protein
- Family history of coronary artery disease
- Hyperlipidemia
- Hypertension
- Hypovolemia
- Hypoxemia
- Hypoxia
- Lack of knowledge of modifiable risk factors (e.g., smoking, sedentary lifestyle, obesity)
- Cardiac surgery
- Cardiac tamponade
- Coronary artery spasm
- Diabetes mellitus

### OUTCOME

#### Cardiac Circulation

- Blood pressure, heart rate, and skin color within normal limits

## Risk for Ineffective Gastrointestinal Perfusion* (2008)

### DEFINITION

At risk for decrease in gastrointestinal circulation

### RISK FACTORS

- Abdominal aortic aneurysm
- Abdominal compartment syndrome
- Abnormal partial thromboplastin time
- Abnormal prothrombin time
- Acute gastrointestinal bleed
- Acute gastrointestinal hemorrhage
- Age > 60 years
- Anemia
- Coagulopathy (e.g., sickle cell anemia)
- Diabetes mellitus
- Disseminated intravascular coagulation
- Female gender
- Gastric paresis (e.g., diabetes mellitus)
- Gastroesophageal varices
- Gastrointestinal disease (e.g., duodenal or gastric ulcer, ischemic colitis, ischemic pancreatitis)
- Hemodynamic instability
- Liver dysfunction
- Myocardial infarction
- Poor left ventricular performance
- Renal failure

### OUTCOME

#### Circulation

- Adequate blood flow to gastrointestinal tissues
- Stroke

*Continues*

*Risk factors require medical intervention or are not changeable (e.g., age, gender); refer to physician.

### Risk for Ineffective Gastrointestinal Perfusion (2008)—*cont'd*

- Trauma
- Smoking
- Treatment-related side effects (e.g., cardiopulmonary bypass, medication, anesthesia, gastric surgery)
- Vascular disease (e.g., peripheral vascular disease, aortoiliac occlusive disease)

**OUTCOME**

**Circulation**

- Adequate blood flow to gastrointestinal tract

## Risk for Ineffective Renal Perfusion (2008)

### DEFINITION

At risk for a decrease in blood circulation to the kidney that may compromise health

### RISK FACTORS*

- Smoking
- Exposure to toxins
- Infection (e.g., sepsis, localized infection)
- Abdominal compartment syndrome
- Advanced age
- Bilateral cortical necrosis
- Burns
- Cardiac surgery
- Cardiopulmonary bypass
- Diabetes mellitus
- Female glomerulonephritis
- Hyperlipidemia
- Hypertension
- Hypovolemia
- Hypoxemia
- Hypoxia
- Malignancy
- Malignant hypertension
- Metabolic acidosis
- Multitrauma
- Polynephritis
- Renal artery stenosis
- Renal disease (e.g., polycystic kidney)
- Systemic inflammatory response syndrome

*Continues*

*Risk factors require medical intervention or are not changeable (e.g., age, gender); refer to physician.

## Risk for Ineffective Renal Perfusion (2008)—*cont'd*

+ Treatment-related side effects (e.g., medications)
+ Vascular embolism vasculitis

**OUTCOME**

**Circulation**

+ Adequate renal blood flow

## Risk for Ineffective Cerebral Tissue Perfusion (2008)

### DEFINITION

Risk for decrease in cerebral tissue circulation

### RISK FACTORS*

- Abnormal partial thromboplastin time
- Abnormal prothrombin time
- Akinetic left ventricular segment
- Aortic atherosclerosis
- Arterial dissection
- Atrial fibrillation
- Atrial myxoma
- Brain tumor
- Carotid stenosis
- Cerebral aneurysm
- Coagulopathy (e.g., sickle cell anemia)
- Dilated cardiomyopathy
- Disseminated intravascular coagulation
- Embolism
- Head trauma
- Hypercholesterolemia
- Left atrial appendage thrombosis
- Hypertension
- Infective endocarditis
- Mechanical prosthetic valve
- Mitral stenosis
- Neoplasm of the brain
- Recent myocardial infarction
- Sick sinus syndrome
- Substance abuse
- Thrombolytic therapy

*Continues*

*Risk factors require medical intervention; refer to physician.

**Risk for Ineffective Cerebral Tissue Perfusion (2008)**—*cont'd*

 • Treatment-related side effects (e.g., cardiopulmonary bypass, medications)

## OUTCOME

### Circulation

 • Adequate blood flow to cerebral tissues

## Autonomic Dysreflexia (1988)

### DEFINITION

Life-threatening uninhibited sympathetic nervous system response to a noxious stimulus with a spinal cord injury of T7 or above

### DEFINING CHARACTERISTICS

#### Diagnostic Cues

- Spinal cord injury (T7 or above)

and one or more of the following:

- Paroxysmal hypertension (sudden, periodic elevated blood pressure; systolic pressure over 140 mm Hg and diastolic 90 mm Hg)
- Diaphoresis (above the injury)
- Headache (a diffuse pain in different portions of the head; not confined to any nerve distribution area)
- Bradycardia or tachycardia (pulse rate of 60 or 100 beats per minute)
- Red splotches on skin (above the injury); pallor below the injury
- Chilling; pilomotor reflex (gooseflesh formation when skin is cooled)
- Paresthesia, blurred vision
- Conjunctival congestion, nasal congestion
- Horner's syndrome (contraction of the pupil, partial ptosis of the eyelid, enophthalmos, sometimes loss of sweating over the affected side of the face)
- Metallic taste in mouth
- Chest pain

*Continues*

## Autonomic Dysreflexia (1988)—*cont'd*

**OUTCOME**

**Neurological Status: Autonomic**

- Normal physiological, autonomic nervous system coordination of visceral and homeostatic function

**HIGH-RISK POPULATIONS**

- Spinal cord injury

**ETIOLOGICAL OR RELATED FACTORS**

- Bladder distention
- Bowel distention
- Skin irritation

## Risk for Autonomic Dysreflexia (1998, 2000)

**DEFINITION**

Risk for life-threatening, uninhibited response of the sympathetic nervous system with spinal cord lesion at T6 or above (after spinal shock); has been demonstrated in patients with injuries at T7 or T8

**RISK FACTORS**

Injury or lesion at T6 and at least one of the following noxious stimuli

**Physiological Factors**

- Bladder distention, spasm
- Catheterization
- Epididymitis, urethritis, urinary tract infection
- Constipation, enemas, stimulation (digital, instrumentation)
- Painful or irritating stimuli below level of injury
- Gastrointestinal pathology (e.g., gastric ulcers, esophageal reflux)
- Bowel distention
- Constipation, fecal impaction
- Digital stimulation; enemas
- Suppositories
- Hemorrhoids
- Temperature fluctuations
- Menstruation, sexual intercourse, ejaculation
- Cutaneous stimuli (pressure ulcer, ingrown toenail, dressings, burns, rash), heterotrophic bone

*Continues*

**Risk for Autonomic Dysreflexia (1998, 2000)—*cont'd***

## Situational Factors

- ◆ Positioning, range-of-motion exercises, pregnancy, labor and delivery, drug reactions (decongestants, sympathomimetics, vasoconstrictors, narcotic withdrawal)
- ◆ Constrictive clothing
- ◆ Fractures
- ◆ Deep-vein thrombosis
- ◆ Ovarian cyst
- ◆ Surgical procedures

## OUTCOME

### Risk Control: Dysreflexia

- ◆ Personal actions are used to prevent, eliminate, or reduce modifiable health threat

## Risk for Sudden Infant Death Syndrome (2002)

### DEFINITION
Presence of risk factors for sudden death of an infant

### RISK FACTORS

#### Modifiable Factors
- Infants placed to sleep in the prone or side lying position
- Prenatal and/or postnatal infant smoke exposure
- Infant overheating/overwrapping
- Soft underlayment/loose articles in the sleep environment
- Delayed or no prenatal care
- Respiratory infection

#### Potentially Modifiable Factors
- Low birth weight
- Prematurity
- Young maternal age

#### Nonmodifiable Factors
- Male gender
- Ethnicity (e.g., African American or Native American race of mother)
- Seasonality of SIDS deaths (higher in winter and fall months)
- SIDS mortality peaks between infant age of 2 to 4 months

### OUTCOME

#### Parenting: Infant/Toddler Physical Safety
- Avoidance of crib injury of a child from birth through 2 years of age

## Disorganized Infant Behavior (1994, 1998)

### DEFINITION

Disintegrated physiological and neurobehavioral responses to the environment

### DEFINING CHARACTERISTICS

#### Physiological/Regulatory System

- Irritability
- Inability to inhibit autonomic system
  - Heart rate (e.g., bradycardia, tachycardia, arrhythmias)
  - Respiratory rate (e.g., bradypnea, tachypnea, apnea)
  - Color (e.g., pale, cyanotic, mottled, flushed)
- Oximeter desaturation
- Feeding intolerance (e.g., aspiration or emesis)
- "Time-out signals" (e.g., gaze, grasp, hiccough, cough, sneeze, yawn, sigh, slack jaw, open mouth, tongue thrust)
- Malnutrition
- Feeding intolerance

#### Motor System

- Increased or decreased muscle tone; limpness
- Tremors, startles, twitches; jittery, jerky, uncoordinated movement
- Hyperextension of arms and legs, finger splay, fisting or hands to face, altered primitive reflexes

#### State-Organization System

- Sleep is diffuse or unclear, state oscillation
- Quiet-awake (staring, gaze aversion)
- Active-awake (fussy, worried gaze)
- Irritable or panicky crying

# ACTIVITY–EXERCISE PATTERN

## Attention-Interaction System

- Abnormal response to sensory stimuli (e.g., difficult to soothe; inability to sustain alert state)

## OUTCOME

### Preterm Infant Organization

- Extrauterine integration of physiologic and behavioral function by the infant born 24- to 37 (term)-weeks gestation

## ETIOLOGICAL OR RELATED FACTORS

- Pain
- Oral or motor problems
- Invasive or painful procedure
- Caregiver factors
- Cue misreading
- Knowledge deficit (cues)
- Environmental stimulation

## HIGH-RISK POPULATIONS

- Prenatal: congenital or genetic disorders, teratogenic exposure
- Postnatal: prematurity
- Individual factors: gestational age, postconceptual age
- Immature neurological system, illness

## Risk for Disorganized Infant Behavior (1994)

### DEFINITION

Risk for disintegration of physiological and neurobehavioral responses to the environment

### RISK FACTORS

- Pain
- Oral or motor problems
- Environmental overstimulation
- Lack of containment or boundaries
- Invasive or painful procedures

### OUTCOME

### Preterm Infant Organization

- Extrauterine integration of physiologic and behavioral function by the infant born 24- to 37 (term)-weeks gestation

## Readiness for Enhanced Organized Infant Behavior (1994)

### DEFINITION

Pattern of modulation of the physiological and functional behavioral systems of an infant (i.e., autonomic, motor, state, organizational, self-regulatory, and attentional–interactional systems) that is satisfactory but that can be improved, resulting in higher levels of integration in response to environmental stimuli

### DEFINING CHARACTERISTICS

- ♦ Stable physiological measures
- ♦ Definite sleep–wake states
- ♦ Use of some self-regulatory behaviors
- ♦ Response to visual or auditory stimuli

### OUTCOME

### Child Development: 1 Month

- ♦ Milestones of physical, cognitive, and psychosocial progression met by 1 month of age

### ETIOLOGICAL OR RELATED FACTORS

- ♦ Prematurity
- ♦ Pain

## ACTIVITY–EXERCISE PATTERN

### Risk for Peripheral Neurovascular Dysfunction* (1992)

**DEFINITION**

Presence of risk factors for disruption in circulation, sensation, or motion of an extremity

**RISK FACTORS**

- Immobilization
- Mechanical compression (e.g., tourniquet, cast or brace, dressing or restraint)
- Orthopedic surgery
- Trauma
- Burns
- Vascular obstruction
- Fractures

**OUTCOME**

**Neurovascular Status**

- Circulation, sensation and motion of extremity intact

---

*Diagnosis encompasses three foci (nutrient supply to tissues, sensation, and motion); thus, it can be viewed as a potentially dysfunctional nutritional–metabolic, perceptual, or activity pattern.

## ACTIVITY–EXERCISE PATTERN

### Decreased Intracranial Adaptive Capacity (1994)

## DEFINITION

Repeated disproportionate increases in intracranial pressure in response to noxious and nonnoxious stimuli caused by lack of compensation for increases in intracranial volumes by intracranial fluid dynamic mechanisms

## DEFINING CHARACTERISTICS

- ◆ Repeated increases of 10 mm Hg for more than 5 minutes following external stimulus
- ◆ Baseline intracranial pressure 10 mm Hg
- ◆ Disproportionate increase in intracranial pressure following single environmental stimulus (e.g., nursing maneuver)
- ◆ Elevated P2 intracranial pressure waveform
- ◆ Volume–pressure response test variation (volume/pressure ratio 2, pressure/volume index 10)
- ◆ Wide-amplitude intracranial pressure waveform

## OUTCOME

### Neurological Status: Consciousness

- ◆ Arousal, orientation, and attention to the environment present

## ETIOLOGICAL OR RELATED FACTORS

- ◆ Decreased cerebral perfusion 50–60 mm Hg
- ◆ Sustained increase in intracranial pressure of 10–15 mm Hg
- ◆ Systemic hypotension with intracranial hypertension

## HIGH-RISK POPULATIONS

- ◆ Brain injuries

## NOTES

**NOTES**

**NOTES**

# Sleep–Rest Pattern

## Insomnia* (1980, 1998)

### DEFINITION

Disruption in amount and quality of sleep that impairs functioning

### DEFINING CHARACTERISTICS

### Diagnostic Cues

- Verbal complaints of not feeling well rested

and one or more of the following:

- Reports interrupted sleep pattern, frequent interruptions during sleep
- Verbal complaints of difficulty falling asleep (delayed sleep onset)
- Sleep pattern reversal

### Supporting Cues

- Reports fatigue
- Reduction in performance (work, school, home)
- Increasing irritability, restlessness
- Early awakening
- Frequent yawning, lethargy
- Dark circles under eyes
- Disorientation (progressive)
- Listlessness
- Expressionless face
- Thick speech with mispronunciation and incorrect words
- Ptosis of eyelids

*Previously titled disturbed sleep pattern. Diagnosis is very broad. See other diagnoses: interrupted sleep pattern, sleep-pattern reversal, delayed sleep onset, and sleep deprivation.

- Mild, fleeting nystagmus
- Slight hand tremor
- Hallucinations, delirium, paranoia

## OUTCOME

### Sleep

- Reports a pattern of feeling well rested after sleep (natural periodic suspension of consciousness for body restoration)

## ETIOLOGICAL OR RELATED FACTORS

- Ruminative (over and over) presleep thoughts
- Physical discomfort (specify)
- Family stress
- Environmental or habit changes (social cues)
- Frequently changing sleep–wake schedule (e.g., shift changes)
- Daytime boredom, inactivity
- Fear (specify)
- Depression
- Anxiety (personal stress)
- Pain
- Perceived vulnerability to harm
- Nocturia
- Sustained use of antisleep agents

## HIGH-RISK POPULATIONS

- Round-the-clock therapy (e.g., treatment/medication required during normal sleep time)
- Nocturnal dyspnea

## Sleep Deprivation (1998)

### DEFINITION
Prolonged periods of time (2 to 3 days or more) without sleep (sustained natural, periodic suspension of relative unconsciousness)

### DEFINING CHARACTERISTICS
#### Diagnostic Cues

- Verbal report of not feeling well rested
- Report of less than usual hours of sleep for 2 to 3 days or more (confirmed, if possible)

and one or more of the following:

- Mood changes
- Restlessness, irritability, anxiety
- Fatigue, lethargy, daytime drowsiness
- Inability to concentrate
- Inability to concentrate, progressing to deterioration in mental and physical task performance and disorientation
- Perceptual disorders (e.g., disturbed body sensation, delusions, feeling afloat, hallucinations, acute confusion)
- Transient paranoia, agitated or combative
- Mild fleeting nystagmus, hand tremors

### OUTCOME
#### Sleep

- Reports a pattern of feeling well rested after sleep (natural periodic suspension of consciousness for body restoration)

## ETIOLOGICAL OR RELATED FACTORS

- Sleep interruptions (specify, e.g., environmental noise)
- Sustained, unfamiliar or uncomfortable sleep environment)
- Depression
- Anxiety; nightmares, sleep terror (children)
- Fear (specify) or vigilance
- Pain-management deficit
- Drugs (that interfere with sleep)
- Presleep activity or work
- Job stress, frequent shift changes
- Age-related sleep stage shifts
- Inadequate daytime activity
- Non–sleep-inducing parenting practices
- Sleep apnea
- Periodic limb movement (e.g., restless leg syndrome, nocturnal myoclonus)
- Sundowners syndrome
- Sleep walking
- Sleep-related painful erections

## Delayed Sleep Onset

### DEFINITION
Inability to sleep when the expectation is that sleep will occur

### DEFINING CHARACTERISTICS
#### Diagnostic Cues
+ Repeated verbal reports of inability to fall asleep after 30 to 45 minutes of expectation that sleep will occur

#### Supporting Cues
+ Reports of not feeling well rested
+ Irritability
+ Fatigue
+ Progressing to inability to concentrate, disorientation, and deterioration in mental and physical task performance

### OUTCOME
#### Sleep
+ Reports a pattern of feeling well rested after sleep (natural periodic suspension of consciousness for body restoration)

### ETIOLOGICAL OR RELATED FACTORS
+ Anxiety
+ Fear (specify)
+ Pain-management deficit
+ Drugs
+ Presleep activity or work
+ Job stress
+ Frequent shift changes

264

## Sleep–Pattern Reversal

### DEFINITION
Change in sleep–wake cycle from nighttime sleep to predominantly daytime sleep

### DEFINING CHARACTERISTICS
#### Diagnostic Cues
- Frequent sleep periods and napping during daytime combined with inability to sleep at night
- Alert during nighttime hours (may engage in activities)

#### Supporting Cues
- Mood changes
- Nocturnal irritability

### OUTCOME
#### Sleep
- Reports a pattern of feeling well rested after sleep (natural periodic suspension of consciousness for body restoration)

### ETIOLOGICAL OR RELATED FACTORS
- Low daytime physical activity or exercise level
- Diversional activity deficit
- Fear or vigilance

### HIGH-RISK POPULATIONS
- Older
- Work shift changes

## Interrupted Sleep Pattern*

### DEFINITION

Time-limited interruptions of sleep amount and quality (caused by external factors)

### DEFINING CHARACTERISTICS

#### Diagnostic Cues

+ Reports being awakened by external factors
+ Change in normal sleep pattern
+ Verbal complaints of not feeling well rested

#### Supporting Cues

+ Dissatisfaction with sleep
+ Decreased ability to function
+ Reports no difficulty falling asleep

### OUTCOME

#### Sleep

+ Reports a pattern of feeling well rested after sleep (natural periodic suspension of consciousness for body restoration)

### ETIOLOGICAL OR RELATED FACTORS

+ Ambient temperature
+ Caregiving responsibilities
+ Change in daylight–darkness exposure
+ Interruptions (e.g., for therapeutics, monitoring, lab tests)
+ Lack of sleep—privacy/control

---

*NANDA-I uses the term *Disturbed Sleep Pattern* for this condition.

## SLEEP–REST PATTERN

- Lighting
- Noise
- Noxious odors
- Physical restraint
- Sleep partner
- Unfamiliar sleep furnishings

## Readiness for Enhanced Sleep (2002)

### DEFINITION

Pattern of natural, periodic, suspension of consciousness that provides adequate rest, sustains a desired lifestyle, and can be strengthened

### Defining Characteristics

- Expresses willingness to enhance sleep
- Amount of sleep and REM sleep is congruent with developmental needs
- Expresses a feeling of being rested after sleep
- Follows sleep routines that promote sleep habits
- Occasional or infrequent use of medications to induce sleep

### OUTCOME

### Sleep

- Reports a pattern of feeling well rested after sleep (natural periodic suspension of consciousness for body restoration)

## NOTES

## NOTES

# Cognitive–Perceptual
# Pattern

## Acute Pain (Specify Type and Location) (1978, 1996, 2002)

### DEFINITION

Verbal or coded report of the presence of indicators of severe discomfort (pain) with a duration of less than 6 months; specify type and location (joint pain, low back, cervical, knee pain)

### DEFINING CHARACTERISTICS

#### Diagnostic Cues

♦ Report of severe discomfort (pain)

and one or more of the following:

- ♦ Guarding behavior, protecting area
- ♦ Muscle tension increased
- ♦ Facial mask of pain (eyes lack luster, "beaten look," fixed or scattered movement, grimace)
- ♦ Restless, irritable
- ♦ Autonomic responses not seen in chronic, stable pain (diaphoresis, blood pressure and pulse rate change, pupillary dilation, increased or decreased respiratory rate)
- ♦ Distraction behavior (moaning, crying, pacing, seeking out other people and/or activities, restless)
- ♦ Focus on self
- ♦ Narrowed focus (altered time perception, withdrawal from social contact, impaired thought process)
- ♦ Listless to rigid; antalgic positioning to avoid pain

### OUTCOME

#### Pain Level

- ♦ Severity: Absence of pain reports

# COGNITIVE–PERCEPTUAL PATTERN

## ETIOLOGICAL OR RELATED FACTORS

+ Knowledge deficit (pain management)

## HIGH-RISK POPULATIONS

+ Postsurgical (e.g., incisional pain)
+ Arthritis (e.g., joint pain)
+ Cardiac (e.g., chest pain)
+ Injuring agents (biological, chemical, physical,
  psychological-stress related); posttrauma, postinjury

## Chronic Pain (Specify Type and Location) (1986, 1996)

### DEFINITION

Severe discomfort (pain) with a duration of more than 6 months; specify type and location (joint pain, low back, cervical, knee pain)

### DEFINING CHARACTERISTICS

#### Diagnostic Cues

- Verbal report or observed evidence of severe discomfort (pain)
- Severe discomfort (pain) experienced for more than 6 months

and one or more of the following:

- Guarded movement
- Altered ability to continue previous activities
- Fear of reinjury
- Facial mask (of pain)
- Physical and social withdrawal
- Anorexia
- Weight changes
- Delayed sleep onset, sleep deprivation

### OUTCOME

#### Pain Level

- Severity: absence of pain reports

### ETIOLOGICAL OR RELATED FACTORS

- Knowledge deficit (chronic pain management)

### HIGH-RISK POPULATIONS

- Chronic physical, psychosocial disability (specify; e.g., cancer)

### Ineffective Pain Self-Management (Chronic, Acute)

**DEFINITION**

Lack of use, or insufficient use, of techniques to reduce pain (e.g., pain medication requests, timing, positioning, distraction)

**DEFINING CHARACTERISTICS**

**Diagnostic Cues**

- Communication (verbal or coded) of pain descriptors
- Delayed requests for medication, lack of use of positioning, distraction, and other pain-management techniques

and one or more of the following:

- Guarding behavior, protecting area
- Self-focusing
- Narrowed focus of attention (e.g., altered time perception, withdrawal from social contact, impaired thought process)
- Distraction behavior (moaning, crying, pacing, seeking out other people and/or activities, restless)
- Facial mask of pain (eyes lack luster, "beaten look," fixed or scattered movement, grimace)
- Muscle tone listless to rigid

**OUTCOME**

- Employs pain management techniques
- Severity: absence of pain reports

**ETIOLOGICAL OR RELATED FACTORS**

- Insufficient knowledge (specify)

*Continues*

**Ineffective Pain Self-Management (Chronic, Acute)—*cont'd***

## HIGH-RISK POPULATIONS

+ Postsurgical (e.g., incisional pain; phantom pain)
+ Arthritis (e.g., joint pain)
+ Cardiac (e.g., chest pain)
+ Injuring agents (biological, chemical, physical, psychological-stress related)
+ Posttrauma

## Impaired Comfort (2009)

### DEFINITION

Perceived lack of ease, relief and transcendence in physical, psychospiritual, environmental, and social dimensions

### DEFINING CHARACTERISTICS

- Anxiety
- Crying
- Disturbed sleep pattern
- Fear
- Illness-related symptoms (see acute pain or pain self-management if pain causing discomfort)
- Inability to relax
- Insufficient resources (e.g., financial, social support)
- Irritability, restlessness
- Lack of environmental control
- Lack of privacy
- Lack of situational control
- Moaning
- Reports being uncomfortable
- Reports being cold or hot
- Reports distressing symptoms
- Reports hunger
- Reports itching
- Reports lack of contentment in situation
- Reports lack of ease in situation

### OUTCOME

#### Comfort Level

- Perceived physical and/or psychosocial ease

### ETIOLOGICAL OR RELATED FACTORS

- Noxious environmental stimuli
- Treatment-related side effects (e.g., medication, radiation)

## Readiness for Enhanced Comfort (2007)

### DEFINITION

A pattern of ease, relief, and transcendence in physical, psychospiritual, environmental, and/or social dimensions that can be strengthened

### DEFINING CHARACTERISTICS

- Expresses desire to enhance comfort
- Expresses desire to enhance feeling of contentment
- Expresses desire to enhance relaxation
- Expresses desire to enhance resolution of complaints

### OUTCOME

- Reports feeling of comfort

## COGNITIVE–PERCEPTUAL PATTERN

### Uncompensated Sensory Loss (Specify Type/Degree)*

**DEFINITION**

Uncompensated decrease in visual, hearing, touch, smell, or kinesthetic acuity (specify degree of loss)

**DEFINING CHARACTERISTICS**

**Diagnostic Cues**

*Vision*

♦ Inability to read newsprint or identify objects and persons

*Hearing*

♦ Inability to identify whispered sounds or normally voiced words

*Touch*

♦ Inability to discriminate various qualities or tactile sensations or absence of tactile perception

*Smell*

♦ Inability to identify odors

*Kinesthesia*

♦ Inability to identify extent, direction, or weight of movement of body or body part

**OUTCOME**

♦ Employs compensation(s) for sensory loss (when cure not possible)

*This condition is frequently a focus for intervention (i.e., an etiological/related factor).

## COGNITIVE–PERCEPTUAL PATTERN

### Sensory Overload

#### DEFINITION
Environmental stimuli greater than habitual level of input and/or monotonous environmental stimuli

#### DEFINING CHARACTERISTICS
#### Diagnostic Cues
- Perceptual distortions of sensory stimuli
- Amount or complexity of sensory stimuli exceeds the usual or desired level (periodic or continuous)
- Presence of uninterrupted intense and/or unchanging stimuli (motor, monitor, light, voices)

#### Supporting Cues
- Reduction in reasoning, problem solving ability, and/or work performance
- Reports sleep disturbances, nightmares
- Disorientation (periodic or general)
- Short attention span
- Restlessness, increased muscle tension
- Reports fatigue
- Irritability, anxiety
- Reports feelings of loss of control

#### OUTCOME
- Reports desired level of sensory stimuli

#### ETIOLOGICAL OR RELATED FACTORS
- Environmental complexity or monotony

#### HIGH-RISK POPULATIONS
- Decreased cognitive capability (e.g., head injury)
- Decreased stress tolerance
- Intensive care monitoring

# COGNITIVE–PERCEPTUAL PATTERN

## Sensory Deprivation

### DEFINITION
Reduced environmental and social stimuli relative to habitual (or basic orienting) level

### DEFINING CHARACTERISTICS
#### Diagnostic Cues
- Amount of sensory stimuli less than usual or desired levels (auditory, visual, proprioceptive, reality-orienting, time-orienting input)
- Disorientation or confusion (periodic, general, nocturnal)

and/or

- Hallucinations, delirium, paranoia

#### Supporting Cues
- Apathy
- Anxiety

### OUTCOME
- Reports desired level of sensory stimuli

### ETIOLOGICAL OR RELATED FACTORS
- Isolation (restricted environment)
- Therapeutic environmental restriction (specify isolation, intensive care, bed rest, traction, confining illness, incubator)
- Socially restricted environment (specify institutionalization, homebound, age debilitation, infant deprivation)
- Uncompensated visual or hearing deficit
- Impaired verbal communication

*Continues*

### Sensory Deprivation—*cont'd*

## HIGH-RISK POPULATIONS

- Congenital or acquired sensory loss
- Social isolation
- Therapeutic isolation

COGNITIVE–PERCEPTUAL PATTERN

## Unilateral Neglect* (1986)

### DEFINITION

Perceptually unaware of and inattentive to one side of the body

### DEFINING CHARACTERISTICS

#### Diagnostic Cues

- Lack of positioning and/or safety precautions in regard to the affected side
- Consistent inattention to stimuli on the affected side
- Does not look toward affected side; ignores objects on affected side
- Leaves food on plate on the affected side

#### Supporting Cues

- Inadequate self-care of affected side

### OUTCOME

#### Adaptation to Physical Disability

- Adaptive response to significant functional challenge due to a physical disability

### HIGH-RISK POPULATIONS

- Cerebrovascular accident (stroke) or other neurological illness/trauma
- One-sided blindness

*This condition is frequently a focus for intervention (i.e., etiological/related factor).

## Deficient Knowledge (Specify Area)* (1980)

### DEFINITION

Inability to state or explain information or demonstrate a required skill related to disease-management procedures, practices, and/or self-care health management (specify area of knowledge deficit, e.g., insulin-dependent diabetic self-care, activity prescription, dietary prescription)

### DEFINING CHARACTERISTICS

#### Diagnostic Cues

- Reports inadequate knowledge
- Inadequate recall, understanding, or misinterpretation, misconception of information,

and one or more of the following:

- Inadequate performance on a test or demonstration of a skill
- Inaccurate responses to questions
- Unable to follow through after instruction

#### Supporting Cues

- Requests information
- Does not comply with prescribed health behaviors
- Inappropriate or exaggerated behaviors (e.g., hysterical, hostile, agitated, apathetic)

### OUTCOME

#### Knowledge

- On request, states cognitive information

---

*This condition is frequently a focus for intervention (i.e., an etiological/related factor).

# COGNITIVE–PERCEPTUAL PATTERN

## ETIOLOGICAL OR RELATED FACTORS

- Low readiness for reception of information
  (e.g., anxiety)
- Lack of interest
- Low motivation to learn
- Uncompensated memory loss
- Inability to use materials or information resources
  (e.g., cultural/language differences)
- Unfamiliarity with information resources

## HIGH-RISK POPULATIONS

- New treatment regimens
- Complex treatment regimens
- Temporary or permanent cognitive limitations
  (intellectual)

### Readiness for Enhanced Knowledge (2002)

**DEFINITION**

Presence or acquisition of cognitive information related to a specific topic is sufficient for meeting health-related goals and can be strengthened

#### Defining Characteristics

- ♦ Expresses an interest in learning
- ♦ Explains knowledge of the topic
- ♦ Behaviors congruent with expressed knowledge
- ♦ Describes previous experiences pertaining to the topic

**OUTCOME**

#### Knowledge

- ♦ States, on request, cognitive-based information

## Ineffective Activity (Task) Planning (2008)

### DEFINITION

Inability to prepare for a set of actions fixed in time and under certain conditions

### DEFINING CHARACTERISTICS

#### Diagnostic Cues

- Verbalization of fear, worry, anxieties toward a task to be undertaken
- Failure pattern of behavior
- Lack of planning
- Lack of sequential organization

#### Supporting Characteristics

- Procrastination
- Lack of resources
- Unmet goals for chosen activity

### OUTCOME

#### Activity Planning

- Plans and completes chosen activities

### ETIOLOGICAL OR RELATED FACTORS

- Compromised ability to process information
- Defensive flight behavior when faced with proposed solution
- Hedonism
- Lack of family support
- Lack of friend support
- Unrealistic perception of events
- Unrealistic perception of personal competence

## Disturbed Thought Processes* (1973, 1996)

### DEFINITION

Disruption in cognitive operations or activities (relative to chronological age expectation) (specify type of alteration, as this is a broad taxonomic category)

### DEFINING CHARACTERISTICS

#### Diagnostic Cues

One or more of the following:

- Impaired perception, judgment, decision making
- Impaired attention span; easily distracted
- Impaired ability to grasp ideas (conceptualize) or order ideas (reason and reflection)
- Inappropriate behavior; non–reality-based thinking

#### Supporting Cues

- Impaired recall ability (see uncompensated memory loss)
- Increased self-concern (egocentricity)
- Hypovigilance or hypervigilance

### OUTCOME

#### Cognition

- Demonstrates ability to execute complex mental processes

### ETIOLOGICAL OR RELATED FACTORS

- Sensory overload (environmental complexity)
- Delayed developmental progression
- Severe anxiety or depression

*See also acute/chronic confusion, impaired environmental interpretation syndrome, uncompensated memory loss, impaired memory, risk for cognitive impairment.

## HIGH-RISK POPULATIONS

- ◆ Dementia; Alzheimer's disease
- ◆ Urinary tract infection (older adult)
- ◆ Fluid and/or electrolyte imbalance
- ◆ Head injury
- ◆ Alcohol or drug abuse

### Attention–Concentration Deficit

**DEFINITION**

Inability to sustain a focal awareness

**DEFINING CHARACTERISTICS**

**Diagnostic Cues**

- Unable to attend to a task for any prolonged period (e.g., more than 5 minutes)
- Easily distracted by any stimulation
- Lack of focus

**Supporting Cues**

- Inability to block stimuli
- Increased sensitivity to stimuli
- Restlessness
- Confusion
- Agitation, frustration, and/or anger

**OUTCOME**

**Concentration**

- Demonstrates ability to focus on a specific stimulus

**HIGH-RISK POPULATIONS**

- Brain injured
- Alzheimer's disease

## Acute Confusion (1994, 2006)

### DEFINITION

Abrupt onset of reversible disturbance of consciousness, attention, cognition, and perception that develop over a short period of time

### DEFINING CHARACTERISTICS

- Fluctuation in cognition
- Fluctuation in level of consciousness
- Fluctuation in sleep–wake cycle
- Fluctuation in psychomotor activity
- Increased agitation or restlessness
- Misperceptions
- Lack of motivation to initiate goal-directed behavior
- Lack of motivation to follow through with goal-directed behavior
- Lack of motivation to initiate purposeful behavior
- Lack of motivation to follow through with purposeful behavior
- Hallucinations

### OUTCOME

#### Cognitive Orientation

- Demonstrates ability to identify person, place and time, accurately

### ETIOLOGICAL OR RELATED FACTORS

- Alcohol abuse
- Drug abuse
- Delirium
- Fluctuation in sleep–wake cycle

*Continues*

### Acute Confusion  (1994, 2006)—*cont'd*

## HIGH-RISK POPULATIONS

+ Dementia
+ Over 60 years of age
+ Hospitalized elderly
+ Elderly relocation (e.g., nursing home)

## Risk for Acute Confusion  (2007)

### DEFINITION

At risk for reversible disturbances of consciousness, attention, cognition, and perception that develop over a short period of time

### RISK FACTORS

- Alcohol use
- Decreased mobility
- Decrease restraints
- Dementia
- Fluctuation in sleep–wake cycle
- History of stroke
- Impaired cognition
- Infection
- Male gender
- Medications/drugs: anticholinergics; opioids; psychoactive drugs
- Multiple medications
- Anesthesia
- Diphenhydramine
- Metabolic abnormalities; azotemia
- Decrease hemoglobin
- Dehydration
- Electrolyte imbalances
- Increased blood urea nitrogen/creatinine
- Malnutrition
- Over 60 years of age
- Pain
- Sensory deprivation
- Substance abuse
- Urinary retention

*Continues*

**Risk for Acute Confusion (2007)—*cont'd***

**OUTCOME**

**Orientation**

- Demonstrates ability to identify person, place and time, accurately

# COGNITIVE–PERCEPTUAL PATTERN

## Chronic Confusion (1994)

### DEFINITION

Irreversible long-standing and/or progressive deterioration of intellect and personality, characterized by decreased ability to interpret environmental stimuli and decreased capacity for intellectual thought processes, and manifested by disturbances of memory, orientation, and behavior

### DEFINING CHARACTERISTICS

- Clinical evidence of organic impairment
- Altered interpretation or response to stimuli
- Progressive or long-standing cognitive impairment
- No change in level of consciousness
- Impaired socialization
- Impaired memory (short term, long term)
- Altered personality

### OUTCOME

**Cognition**

- Ability to execute complex mental processes (if no resolution, see Risk for Injury)

### HIGH-RISK POPULATIONS

- Alzheimer's disease
- Korsakoff's psychosis
- Multi-infarct dementia
- Cerebral vascular accident
- Head injury
- Over 60 years of age
- Delirium

# COGNITIVE–PERCEPTUAL PATTERN

## Impaired Environmental Interpretation Syndrome (1994)

### DEFINITION
Consistent lack of orientation to person, place, time, or circumstances over more than 3 to 6 months that necessitates a protective environment

### DEFINING CHARACTERISTICS
- Consistent disorientation in known and unknown environments for more than 3 to 6 months
- Chronic confusional states
- Loss of occupational or social functioning from memory decline
- Inability to follow simple directions, instructions
- Inability to reason
- Inability to concentrate
- Slow in responding to questions

### OUTCOME
#### Cognitive Orientation
- Demonstrates ability to identify person, place and time, accurately

### ETIOLOGICAL OR RELATED FACTORS
- Depression
- Alcoholism

### HIGH-RISK POPULATIONS
- Dementia (Alzheimer's, multi-infarct dementia, Pick's disease, AIDS dementia)
- Parkinson's disease
- Huntington's disease

## COGNITIVE–PERCEPTUAL PATTERN

### Uncompensated Memory Loss

#### DEFINITION
Impaired ability to recall recent events and activities

#### DEFINING CHARACTERISTICS
#### Diagnostic Cues

♦ Frequent episodes of inability to recall recent events, information received, and/or activities, names, places
♦ Lack of use (or unsuccessful use) of devices or procedures to support memory

#### Supporting Cues

♦ Inability to recall previously learned activities, names, places
♦ Begins an activity and unable to recall intention seconds or minutes later
♦ Lack of understanding and problem solving based on deficit in short-term recall (minutes, hours)

#### OUTCOME
#### Memory

♦ Ability cognitively to retrieve and report previously stored information with or without compensation

#### HIGH-RISK POPULATIONS

♦ Alzheimer's disease
♦ Degenerative neurological conditions

## Impaired Memory (1994)

### DEFINITION

Inability to remember or recall bits of information or behavioral skills (impaired memory may be attributed to pathophysiological or situational causes that are either temporary or permanent)

### DEFINING CHARACTERISTICS

- Observed or reported experiences of forgetting
- Inability to determine whether a behavior was performed
- Inability to learn or retain new skills or information
- Inability to perform a previously learned skill
- Inability to recall factual information
- Inability to recall recent or past events
- Forgetting to perform a behavior at a scheduled time

### OUTCOME

#### Memory

- Ability cognitively to retrieve and report previously stored information with or without compensation

### ETIOLOGICAL OR RELATED FACTORS

- Acute or chronic hypoxia
- Anemia
- Decreased cardiac output
- Fluid and electrolyte imbalance
- Neurological disturbances
- Excessive environmental disturbances

## Risk for Cognitive Impairment

### DEFINITION

Presence of risk factors for impairment in memory, reasoning ability, judgment, and decision making

### RISK FACTORS

- Receiving tranquilizers, sedatives
- Low self-initiative in providing cognitive stimulation
- Borderline neurophysiological pathology
- Confinement to environment low in cognitive stimulation (perceptual, problem solving, decision making)
- Hearing and/or vision deficit combined with decreased stimulation and/or relocation

### OUTCOME

### Cognition

- Demonstrates ability to execute complex mental processes

## Readiness for Enhanced Decision Making (2007)

### DEFINITION

Pattern of choosing courses of action that is sufficient for meeting short and long term health-related goals and can be strengthened

### DEFINING CHARACTERISTICS

- Expresses desire to enhance decision making
- Expresses desire to enhance congruency of decisions with personal values and goals
- Expresses desire to enhance congruency of decisions with sociocultural values and goals
- Expresses desire to enhance risk benefit analysis of decisions
- Expresses desire to enhance understanding of choices for decision making
- Expresses desire to enhance understanding of the meaning of choices
- Expresses desire to enhance use of reliable evidence for decisions

### OUTCOME

### Decision Making

- Demonstrates ability to make judgments and choose between two or more alternatives

## Decisional Conflict (Specify) (1988)

### DEFINITION

Uncertainty about course of action to be taken when choice among competing actions involves risk, loss, or challenge to personal life values (specify focus of conflict, e.g., surgery, therapy, abortion, divorce, or other life events)

### DEFINING CHARACTERISTICS

#### Diagnostic Cues

- Delayed decision making and/or vacillation between alternative choices
- Verbalized uncertainty about choices
- Verbalized feeling of distress while attempting a decision
- Physical signs of distress or tension (e.g., increased heart rate, increased muscle tension, or restlessness)

#### Supporting Cues

- Verbalization of undesired consequences of alternative actions being considered
- Questioning personal values and beliefs while attempting to make a decision
- Self-focusing

### OUTCOME

#### Decision Making

- Demonstrates ability to make judgments and choose between two or more alternatives

*Continues*

## Decisional Conflict (Specify) (1988)—*cont'd*

### ETIOLOGICAL OR RELATED FACTORS

- Perceived threat to value system
- Unclear personal values or beliefs
- Lack of experience or interference with decision making; lack of relevant information; multiple or divergent information sources
- Support system deficit

### HIGH-RISK POPULATIONS

- Relocation decisions (e.g., nursing home, moving)
- Terminal illness (treatment preferences)
- Surgical or treatment choices
- Abusive situations

## NOTES

# NOTES

# Self-Perception–
# Self-Concept Pattern

## Fear (Specify Focus)* (1980, 1996, 2000)

### DEFINITION

Feeling of dread related to an identifiable source that is perceived as a threat or danger to the self (specify focus; e.g., prognosis, surgical outcome, death, disability)

### DEFINING CHARACTERISTICS

#### Diagnostic Cues

- Report of feelings of dread, nervousness, or worry/concern about a threatening event, person, or object with expectation of danger to the self
- Describes (with or without assistance) the focus of perceived threat or danger (potential, actual, or imagined)
- Narrowing focus of attention progressing to fixed (increased severity)

and one or more of the following:

- Restlessness; fidgeting
- Increased questioning or information seeking
- Increased heart rate, increased respiratory rate
- Increased muscle tension
- Increase in quantity or rate of verbalization
- Vigilance/scanning surroundings
- Voice tremors, pitch changes
- Hand tremor
- Diaphoresis
- Diminished productivity
- Irritability

*This condition is frequently a focus for intervention (i.e., etiological/related factor).

## SELF-PERCEPTION–SELF-CONCEPT PATTERN

**Severe**

- Anguish
- Uncertainty
- Distress
- Sleep disturbance
- Confusion (older persons)

## OUTCOME

**Fear**

- Absence of apprehension, tension, or uneasiness from an identifiable source

## ETIOLOGICAL OR RELATED FACTORS

- Knowledge deficit/unfamiliarity with environmental experience(s)
- Perceived inability to control events (see powerlessness)
- Language barrier
- Sensory impairment (specify)
- Phobic stimulus

## HIGH-RISK POPULATIONS

- Surgical or diagnostic procedures
- Surgical outcome
- First hospitalization
- Discharge to self-care
- Support system deficit (in stressful situation)

## SELF-PERCEPTION–SELF-CONCEPT PATTERN

### Anxiety (1973, 1982, 1998)

#### DEFINITION
Vague, uneasy feeling of discomfort or dread, the source of which is often nonspecific or unknown to the individual

#### DEFINING CHARACTERISTICS

#### Diagnostic Cues

+ Reports feeling "anxious," apprehensive, tense, scared, worried, "fearful"
+ Reports vague, uneasy feeling of concern about unspecified consequences or changes in life events

and one or more of the following:

+ Reports inability to relax, feeling jittery
+ Increased muscle tension, foot shuffling, hand or arm movements, trembling, hand tremor, shakiness
+ Facial tension
+ Lack of concentration
+ Insomnia
+ Sympathetic response (increased heart rate, respiratory rate, dilated pupils)

#### Supporting Cues

+ Focus on self
+ Verbalizes painful and persistent feelings of increased helplessness, inadequacy, regret (see also Ineffective Coping)
+ Restlessness, fidgeting, increased perspiration
+ Overexcited, rattled, jittery, scared
+ Increased wariness, glancing about, poor eye contact, facial tension, voice quivering

- Diminished productivity
- Scanning the environment, vigilance, impaired attention
- Irritability, anguish, distress

## OUTCOME

### Anxiety Level

- Absence of apprehension, tension, or uneasiness from an unidentifiable source

## ETIOLOGICAL OR RELATED FACTORS

- Perceived threat to self-concept, health status, socioeconomic status, role functioning, interaction patterns, or environment
- Unconscious conflict (essential values or life goals)
- Unmet needs (specify)
- Interpersonal transmission or contagion
- Uncertainty

## Mild Anxiety

### DEFINITION

Increased level of arousal associated with expectation of a threat (unfocused) to the self or significant relationships

### DEFINING CHARACTERISTICS

- Verbalizes feelings of increased arousal, concern, vigilance
- Increased questioning
- Increased awareness
- Increased attending
- Mild restlessness
- Lip chewing, nail biting, foot movements, finger or pencil tapping

### OUTCOME

**Anxiety Level**

- Absence of apprehension, tension, or uneasiness from an unidentifiable source

### ETIOLOGICAL OR RELATED FACTORS

- Perceived threat to self-concept, health status, socioeconomic status, role functioning, interaction patterns, or environment
- Unconscious conflict (essential values or life goals)
- Unmet needs (specify)
- Interpersonal transmission or contagion

## Moderate Anxiety

### DEFINITION

Increased level of arousal with selective attention and associated with expectation of a threat (unfocused) to the self or significant relationships

### DEFINING CHARACTERISTICS

- Expressed feelings of unfocused apprehension, nervousness, or concern
- Verbalizes expectation of danger
- Voice tremors, pitch changes, hand tremor
- Narrowing focus of attention
- Increased rate of verbalization
- Restlessness, pacing, increased muscle tension
- Diaphoresis
- Increased heart and respiratory rate
- Sleep or eating disturbances

### OUTCOME

#### Anxiety Level

- Absence of apprehension, tension, or uneasiness from an unidentifiable source

### ETIOLOGICAL OR RELATED FACTORS

- Separation (use separation anxiety)
- Perceived threat to self-concept, health status, socioeconomic status, role functioning, interaction patterns, or environment
- Unconscious conflict (essential values or life goals)
- Unmet needs (specify)
- Interpersonal transmission or contagion

## Severe Anxiety (Panic)

### DEFINITION

Extreme arousal and scattered focus associated with expectation of a threat to the self or to significant relationships

### DEFINING CHARACTERISTICS

+ Feelings of unfocused and severe dread, apprehension, nervousness, or concern
+ Inappropriate verbalization or absence of verbalization
+ Diminished ability to problem solve
+ Purposeless activity or immobilization
+ Perceptual focus scattered or fixed or inability to focus on reality
+ Increased heart rate
+ Hyperventilation
+ Diaphoresis
+ Increased muscle tension
+ Dilated pupils
+ Pallor

### OUTCOME

**Anxiety Level**

+ Absence of apprehension, tension, or uneasiness from an unidentifiable source

### ETIOLOGICAL OR RELATED FACTORS

+ Perceived threat to self-concept, health status, socioeconomic status, role functioning, interaction patterns, or environment
+ Unconscious conflict (essential values or life goals)
+ Unmet needs (specify)
+ Interpersonal transmission or contagion

## Anticipatory Anxiety (Mild, Moderate, Severe)

### DEFINITION

Increased level of arousal associated with a perceived future threat (unfocused) to the self or significant relationships

### DEFINING CHARACTERISTICS

#### Diagnostic Cues

- Reports feeling anxious, apprehensive, jittery, tense, or fearful
- Reports vague, uneasy feeling about unspecified future or impending event perceived as a threat to the self or significant relationships (unfocused)

and one or more of the following:

- Inability to relax
- Increased muscle tension, restless, foot shuffling, hand or arm movements, trembling
- Sympathetic response (increased heart rate, respiratory rate, pupils dilated)

### OUTCOME

#### Anxiety Level

- Absence of apprehension, tension, or uneasiness from an unidentifiable source

### ETIOLOGICAL OR RELATED FACTORS

- Perceived threat to self-concept, health status, socioeconomic status, role functioning, interaction patterns, or environment
- Unconscious conflict (essential values or life goals); unmet needs
- Interpersonal transmission or contagion

## Death Anxiety (1998)

### DEFINITION
Vague uneasy feeling of discomfort or dread generated by real or imagined threat to one's existence

### DEFINING CHARACTERISTICS
### Diagnostic Cues

- Expresses deep sadness
- Reports concerns/fears about dying

and one or more of the following:

### Concerns: Others

- Worrying about the impact of own death on significant others (grief and suffering)
- Concerns about overworking the caregiver as terminal illness incapacitates self
- Worrying about being the cause of others' grief and suffering
- Fear of leaving family alone after death

### Concerns: Dying Process

- Expresses "fear" of the process of dying
- Powerlessness (issues related to dying)
- Expresses "fear" of loss of physical and/or mental abilities when dying
- Anticipation of pain related to dying
- Expresses concern over total loss of control over any aspect of own death
- Negative death images or unpleasant thoughts about any event related to death and dying
- Fear of prolonged dying

- Fear of premature death because it prevents the accomplishment of important life goals
- Fear of developing a terminal illness

## Concerns: After Death

- Concern about meeting one's creator or feeling doubtful about the existence of a god or higher being
- Denial of own mortality or impending death
- Uncertainty about life after death

## OUTCOME

### Anxiety Level

- Absence of apprehension, tension, or uneasiness about death/dying process

## ETIOLOGICAL OR RELATED FACTORS

- Diagnosis incorporates probable focus of anxiety/fear, that is, death
- Focus of treatment is on anxiety/fears about death

### Reactive Depression (Specify Focus)

**DEFINITION**

Acute decrease in self-esteem, worth, or competency linked to a situational threat (specify situational threat; e.g., health outcome, disability, physical deterioration)

**DEFINING CHARACTERISTICS**

**Diagnostic Cues**

- Expressions of sadness, despair, or hopelessness about a situation (specify situation)
- Continual questioning of self-worth (self-esteem) or feeling of failure (real or imagined)
- Pessimistic outlook

and one or more of the following to determine severity:

- Withdrawal from others to avoid possible rejection (real or imagined)
- Suspicion or sensitivity to words and actions of others related to general lack of trust of others
- Threats or attempts to commit suicide (refer for immediate evaluation, if observed)
- Extreme dependency on others with related feelings of helplessness and anger
- Misdirected anger (toward self)
- General irritability
- Guilt feelings
- Inability to concentrate on reading, writing, conversation
- Change (usually decrease) in physical activities, eating, sleeping, sexual activity
- Early morning awakening

## SELF-PERCEPTION–SELF-CONCEPT PATTERN

**OUTCOME**

**Depression Level**

- ◆ Absence of melancholic mood
- ◆ Positive expressions of self worth/interest in life events

**ETIOLOGICAL OR RELATED FACTORS**

- ◆ Perceived powerlessness
- ◆ Anxiety

**HIGH-RISK POPULATIONS**

- ◆ Debilitating surgery or trauma, new physical disability
- ◆ Significant personal loss

## SELF-PERCEPTION–SELF-CONCEPT PATTERN

### Risk for Loneliness (1994)

**DEFINITION**

Risk for experiencing vague dysphoria

**RISK FACTORS**

- Feelings of deprivation of affection
- Physical isolation
- Cathectic deprivation
- Social isolation

**OUTCOME**

**Loneliness Severity**

- Absence of expressed feelings of emotional, social, or existential isolation

## Hopelessness* (1986)

### DEFINITION

Perception of limited or no alternatives or personal choices available and unable to mobilize energy on own behalf

### DEFINING CHARACTERISTICS

#### Diagnostic Cues

- Verbalization of despondent or hopeless content (e.g., "I can't," sighing; feel empty, drained; "end of my rope," feeling of deprivation, impossibility)
- Lack of initiative or ambition (e.g., lack of involvement in care; passively allowing care)
- Decreased affect

and one or more of the following:

- General passivity; decreased verbalization
- Decreased appetite
- Increased sleep time
- Shrugging in response to speaker
- Closing eyes
- Turning away from speaker
- Decreased response to stimuli
- Expresses the perception of no alternatives (severe)

### OUTCOME

#### Hope

- Expressions of optimism that is personally satisfying and life supporting

*Continues*

---

*See also Powerlessness, Situational Depression.

## Hopelessness (1986)—*cont'd*

### ETIOLOGICAL OR RELATED FACTORS

+ Prolonged activity restriction (creating isolation)
+ Abandonment
+ Loss of belief (transcendent values or God)

### HIGH-RISK POPULATIONS

+ Impaired adjustment to chronic or terminal illness (self or significant other)
+ Chronic pain
+ Self-care or mobility deficits
+ Activity intolerance
+ History of long-term stress
+ Failing or deteriorating physiological condition
+ Long-term stress

## Readiness for Enhanced Hope (2007)

### DEFINITION

Pattern of expectations and desires that is sufficient for mobilizing energy on one's own behalf and can be strengthened

### DEFINING CHARACTERISTICS

- Expresses desire to enhance ability to set achievable goals
- Expresses desire to enhance belief in possibilities
- Expresses desire to enhance congruency of expectations with desires
- Expresses desire to enhance hope
- Expresses desire to enhance interconnectedness with others
- Expresses desire to enhance problem solving to meet goals
- Expresses desire to enhance sense of meaning to life
- Expresses desire to enhance spirituality

### OUTCOME

#### Hope

- Expressions of optimism that is personally satisfying and life supporting

## Powerlessness (Severe, Moderate, Low)* (1982)

### DEFINITION

Perceived lack of control over a situation and perception that own actions will not significantly affect an outcome

### DEFINING CHARACTERISTICS

### Diagnostic Cues

*Severe*

- ♦ Verbalization of having no control or influence over a situation, an outcome(s), or self-care
- ♦ Does not participate in healthcare decisions
- ♦ Apathy

### Supporting Cues

- ♦ Depressed over physical deterioration despite compliance with regimens

*Moderate*

- ♦ Passivity

and one or more of the following:

- ♦ Expressed doubt regarding role performance
- ♦ Expressed dissatisfaction or frustration over inability to perform previous roles, tasks, activities
- ♦ Dependence on others that may result in irritability, resentment, anger, guilt
- ♦ Nonparticipation in care or decision making when opportunities provided
- ♦ Reluctance to express true feelings fearing alienation from caregivers
- ♦ Does not monitor progress, seek information regarding care, or defend self-care practices when challenged

*See also Reactive Depression, Hopelessness.

# SELF-PERCEPTION–SELF-CONCEPT PATTERN

*Low*

+ Expressed uncertainty about fluctuating energy levels
+ Passivity

## OUTCOME

### Health Beliefs: Perceived Control

+ Personal conviction that one can influence a health/life outcome

## ETIOLOGICAL OR RELATED FACTORS

+ Healthcare environment (specify aspect)
+ Perceived interpersonal control by others
+ Lifestyle of helplessness
+ Impaired verbal communication

## HIGH-RISK POPULATIONS

+ Degenerative disease
+ Forced relocation
+ Institutional residency

## Risk for Powerlessness  (2000)

### DEFINITION

At risk for perceived lack of control over a situation and/or ability to significantly affect an outcome

### RISK FACTORS

#### Physiological

- Chronic or acute illness (hospitalization, intubation, ventilator, suctioning)
- Acute injury or progressive debilitating disease process (e.g., spinal cord injury, multiple sclerosis)
- Aging (e.g., decreased physical strength, decreased mobility)
- Dying

#### Psychosocial

- Lack of knowledge of illness or healthcare system
- Lifestyle of dependency with inadequate coping patterns
- Absence of integrality (e.g., essence of power)
- Decreased self-esteem
- Low or unstable body image

### OUTCOME

#### Health Beliefs: Perceived Control

- Personal conviction that one can influence a health/life outcome

## Readiness for Enhanced Power (2007)

### DEFINITION

Pattern of participating in change that is sufficient for well-being and can be strengthened

### DEFINING CHARACTERISTICS

+ Expresses readiness to enhance awareness of possible changes to be made
+ Expresses readiness to enhance freedom to perform actions for change
+ Expresses readiness to enhance identification of choices that can be made for change
+ Expresses readiness to enhance involvement in creating change
+ Expresses readiness to enhance knowledge for participation in change
+ Expresses readiness to enhance participation in choices for daily living and health
+ Expresses readiness to enhance power

### OUTCOME

### Health Beliefs: Perceived Control

+ Personal conviction that a health/life outcome can be influenced

## Risk for Compromised Human Dignity (2007)

### DEFINITION

Risk for perception of a loss of respect and honor

### RISK FACTORS

- Cultural incongruity
- Disclosure of confidential information
- Exposure of the body
- Inadequate participation in decision making
- Stigmatizing label
- Use of undefined medical terms
- Loss of control of body functions
- Perceived dehumanizing conditions
- Perceived humiliation
- Perceived intrusion by clinicians
- Perceived invasion of privacy

As stated, this may not be a patient diagnosis but rather a care delivery problem. One school of thought is that human dignity is an inherent characteristic. It can be threatened or affronted, but not given up or compromised. Last four characteristics alone may indicate perceived threat to human dignity.

## SELF-PERCEPTION–SELF-CONCEPT PATTERN

### Situational Low Self-Esteem* (1988, 1996, 2000)

#### DEFINITION

Development of a negative perception of self-worth in response to a current situation

#### DEFINING CHARACTERISTICS

#### Diagnostic Cues

- ♦ Repeated self-negating verbalizations (negative feelings about self)
- ♦ Evaluation of self as unable to deal with situations or events

and one or more of the following:

- ♦ Lack of eye contact
- ♦ Head flexion
- ♦ Shoulder flexion

#### Supporting Cues

- ♦ Indecisive; nonassertive
- ♦ Hesitation to try new things or situations
- ♦ Rationalizations or rejections of positive feedback
- ♦ Exaggerations of negative feedback about self
- ♦ Hypersensitivity to a slight or a criticism
- ♦ Expressions of shame or guilt
- ♦ Expressions of helplessness and uselessness
- ♦ Compensations
- ♦ Grandiosity (see also defensive coping)
- ♦ Denial of problems obvious to others (see also defensive coping)

*Continues*

---

*This condition is frequently a focus for intervention (i.e., an etiological/related factor).

## Situational Low Self-Esteem (1988, 1996, 2000)—*cont'd*

+ Projection of blame or responsibility for problems
  (see also defensive coping)
+ Rationalization of personal failures (see also defensive
  coping)

**OUTCOME**

**Self-Esteem**

+ Demonstrates feeling of self-worth and competency

**ETIOLOGICAL OR RELATED FACTORS**

+ Developmental changes (specify)
+ Disturbed body image
+ Functional impairment (specify)
+ Loss (specify)
+ Social role changes (specify)
+ Lack of recognition/rewards
+ Behavior inconsistent with values
+ Failures/rejections

## SELF-PERCEPTION–SELF-CONCEPT PATTERN

### Risk for Situational Low Self-Esteem  (2000)

#### DEFINITION

Presence of risk factors for developing negative perception of self-worth in response to a current situation (specify)

#### RISK FACTORS

- Developmental changes (specify)
- Disturbed body image
- Functional impairment (specify)
- Loss (specify)
- Social role changes (specify)
- Lack of recognition/rewards
- Behavior inconsistent with values
- Failures/rejections
- Unrealistic self-expectations
- History of abuse/neglect/abandonment

#### OUTCOME

#### Self-Esteem

- Demonstrates feeling of self-worth and competency

## Chronic Low Self-Esteem* (1988, 1996, 2008)

### DEFINITION

Long-standing negative self-evaluation/feelings about self or self capabilities

### DEFINING CHARACTERISTICS

#### Diagnostic Cues

All behaviors here are long-standing/chronic:
- Repeated self-negating verbalizations
- Lack of eye contact, head flexion, and/or shoulder flexion

#### Supporting Cues

- Evaluations of self as unable to deal with events
- Hesitation to try new things or situations
- Exaggerations of negative feedback about self
- Rejection of positive feedback about self
- Frequent lack of success in work or other life events
- Overly conforming, dependent on others' opinions
- Nonassertive or passive
- Indecisive behavior
- Excessively seeking reassurance
- Expressions of shame or guilt
- High level of negative criticism from significant other

### OUTCOME

#### Self-Esteem

- Personal feeling/expression of self-worth and competency

---

*This condition is frequently a focus for intervention (e.g., etiological/related factors).

# SELF-PERCEPTION–SELF-CONCEPT PATTERN

## ETIOLOGICAL OR RELATED FACTORS

+ Ineffective adaptation to loss
+ Lack of affection/approval
+ Lack of membership in group; perceived lack of belonging
+ Perceived discrepancy between self and spiritual or cultural norms
+ Perceived lack of respect from others
+ Repeated negative reinforcement from failures
+ Traumatic event or situation

## HIGH-RISK POPULATIONS

+ Psychiatric disorder
+ Repeated failures
+ Total self-care deficit

## Readiness for Enhanced Self-Concept (2002)

### DEFINITION

Pattern of perception or ideas about the self that is sufficient for well-being and can be strengthened

### DEFINING CHARACTERISTICS

- Expresses willingness to enhance self-concept
- Expresses satisfaction with thoughts about self, sense of worthiness, role performance, body image, and personal identity
- Actions are congruent with expressed feelings and thoughts
- Expresses confidence in abilities
- Accepts strengths and limitations

### OUTCOME

**Self-Esteem**

- Consistently demonstrates personal feeling of self-worth and competency

## Disturbed Body Image* (1973, 1998)

### DEFINITION
Negative feelings or perceptions about characteristics, functions, or limits of body or body part

### DEFINING CHARACTERISTICS
#### Diagnostic Cues
- Verbalized actual or perceived change in structure and/or function of body or body part
- Verbalized feelings of helplessness, hopelessness, and/or powerlessness in relation to body and fear of rejection or reaction of others

and one or more of the following:
- Verbalized negative feelings about body (e.g., dirty, big, small, unsightly)
- Repeated expressions of negative feeling about loss of body fluids, addition of body fluids or machines
- Repeated verbalizations focusing on past strength, function, or appearance

#### Supporting Cues
- Verbalized change in lifestyle because of negative feelings or perceptions of body
- Preoccupation with change in body or loss of part
- Refusal to verify actual change in body or body part
- Change in ability to estimate spatial relationship of body to environment
- Personalization of part, or loss, by name
- Depersonalization of part or loss by impersonal pronoun

*Continues*

*This condition is frequently a focus for intervention (e.g., etiological/related factors).

### Disturbed Body Image (1973, 1998)—*cont'd*

- Extension of body boundary to incorporate environmental objects (e.g., machines, oxygen, respirator)
- Emphasis on remaining strengths or heightened achievement
- Trauma to nonfunctioning part (intentional or nonintentional)
- Change in social involvement or social relationships
- Hiding or overexposing body part
- Not touching body part
- Not looking at body part

## OUTCOME

### Body Image

- Positive perception of own appearance and body functions

## ETIOLOGICAL OR RELATED FACTORS

- Nonintegration of change (in body characteristics, function, or limits)
- Perceived developmental imperfections
- Obesity

## HIGH-RISK POPULATIONS

- Hemiplegia
- Loss of a body part (e.g., leg amputation, breast removal)
- Loss or change in body function (e.g., reproductive, elimination)
- Loss of body part
- Facial trauma
- Pacemaker implant
- Congenital anomalies (observable)

### Disturbed Personal Identity (1978, 2008)

#### DEFINITION

Inability to maintain an integrated perception of self or distinguish between self and nonself

#### DEFINING CHARACTERISTICS

#### Diagnostic Cues

One or more of the following:
* Unable to distinguish self from others or objects
* Unable to distinguish between inner and outer stimuli
* Verbalizations of "not knowing who I am;" delusional description of self
* Expresses feelings of emptiness or strangeness
* Gender confusion

#### Supporting Cues

* Disturbed body image
* Disturbed relationships
* Ineffective coping
* Fluctuating feelings about self
* Ineffective role performance
* Uncertainty about goals
* Uncertainty about cultural or ideological values (e.g., beliefs, religion, moral questions)

#### OUTCOME

#### Identity

* Distinguishes between self and nonself

*Continues*

## Disturbed Personal Identity (1978, 2008)—*cont'd*

### ETIOLOGICAL OR RELATED FACTORS

- Use of psychoactive drugs
- Cult indoctrination
- Cultural discontinuity
- Discrimination or prejudice
- Dysfunctional family processes
- Low self-esteem
- Manic states
- Situational crises
- Social role change
- Inhalation or ingestion of toxic chemicals

### HIGH-RISK POPULATIONS

- Multiple personality disorder
- Organic brain syndrome
- Psychiatric disorders (e.g., psychoses, depression, dissociative disorder)
- Stages of growth
- Stages of development

## Risk for Self-Directed Violence (1994)

### DEFINITION

Presence of risk factors for behavior that can be physically, emotionally, and/or sexually harmful to the self

### RISK FACTORS

* Suicidal ideation (frequent, intense, prolonged)
* Suicidal plan (clear and specific lethality; method and availability of destructive means)
* History of multiple suicide attempts; family history of suicide
* Behavioral clues (e.g., writing forlorn love notes, directing angry messages at a significant other who has rejected the person, giving away personal items, taking out a large insurance policy)
* Verbal clues (e.g., talking about death, "better off without me," asking questions about lethal dosages of drugs)
* Emotional status (hopelessness, despair, increased anxiety, panic, anger, hostility)
* Mental health (severe depression, psychosis, severe personality disorder, alcoholism or drug abuse)
* Conflict in interpersonal relationships
* Marital status (single, widowed, divorced)
* Occupation (executive, administrator/owner of business, professional, or semiskilled worker)
* Employment (unemployed, recent job loss/failure)
* Personal resources (poor achievement, poor insight)
* Social resources (poor rapport, socially isolated, unresponsive family)
* Family background (chaotic or conflictual)

*Continues*

### Risk for Self-Directed Violence (1994)—*cont'd*

- Engagement in autoerotic sexual acts
- Age 15 to 19 years and over 45 years
- Sexual orientation (active bisexual, inactive homosexual)

**OUTCOME**

**Suicide Self-Restraint**

- Takes personal actions to refrain from gestures and attempts at killing self

**NOTES**

## NOTES

# Role–Relationship

# Pattern

## Anticipatory Grieving* (1980, 1996)

### DEFINITION

Expectation of disruption/loss in a familiar pattern or significant relationships (includes people, possessions, job, status, home, ideals, body part or body process)

### DEFINING CHARACTERISTICS

#### Diagnostic Cues

+ Potential for loss of significant people, possessions, job, status, home, ideals, and parts and processes of the body
+ Verbal expression of distress at potential (anticipated) loss

and one or more of the following:

+ Anger
+ Sadness, sorrow, crying
+ Crying at frequent intervals, choked feeling
+ Change in eating habits
+ Alteration in sleep or dream patterns
+ Alteration in activity level
+ Altered libido
+ Idealization of anticipated loss
+ Developmental regression
+ Alteration in concentration or pursuit of tasks

### OUTCOME

#### Grief Resolution

+ Adjusts to impending loss

---

*This condition is frequently a focus for intervention (e.g., etiological/related factor).

# ROLE–RELATIONSHIP PATTERN

## Grieving (2006)

### DEFINITION

A normal complex process (emotional, physical, spiritual, social, and intellectual responses/behaviors) by which individuals, families, and communities incorporate an actual, anticipated, or perceived loss into their daily lives

### DEFINING CHARACTERISTICS

#### Diagnostic Cues

- Experience of loss

and one or more of the following:

- Alteration in activity level
- Alterations in immune function
- Alterations in neuroendocrine function
- Alterations in sleep patterns
- Alteration in dream patterns
- Anger
- Blame
- Detachment
- Despair
- Disorganization

#### Supporting Cues

- Maintaining the connection to the deceased
- Making meaning of the loss
- Experiencing relief
- Pain
- Panic behavior
- Personal growth
- Psychological distress
- Suffering

*Continues*

Grieving (2006)—*cont'd*

**OUTCOME**

**Grief Resolution**

 ♦ Adjusts to loss

**ETIOLOGICAL OR RELATED FACTORS**

 ♦ Anticipatory loss if significant object (e.g., possession, job, status, home, parts, and processes of body)
 ♦ Anticipatory loss if a significant other
 ♦ Death of a significant other
 ♦ Loss of significant object (e.g., possession, job, status, home, parts, and processes of body)

## Complicated Grieving  (2006)

### DEFINITION

A disorder that occurs after the death of a significant other, in which the experience of distress accompanying bereavement fails to follow normative expectations and manifests in functional impairment

### DEFINING CHARACTERISTICS

#### Diagnostic Cues

- ♦ Prolonged decrease in functioning (life roles)
- ♦ Decreased sense of well-being
- ♦ Lack of acceptance of the loss, for example, death

and one or more of the following:

- ♦ Depression
- ♦ Experiencing somatic symptoms of the deceased
- ♦ Fatigue
- ♦ Grief avoidance
- ♦ Low levels of intimacy
- ♦ Persistent emotional distress
- ♦ Persistent painful memories
- ♦ Preoccupation with thoughts of the deceased
- ♦ Rumination, longing, and searching for the deceased
- ♦ Separation distress
- ♦ Verbalizes anxiety, distress
- ♦ Verbalizes feeling dazed and empty
- ♦ Verbalizes feeling in shock or stunned
- ♦ Verbalizes feelings of anger and self blame
- ♦ Verbalizes feelings of detachment from others
- ♦ Verbalizes feelings of disbelief
- ♦ Verbalizes feelings of mistrust
- ♦ Yearning

*Continues*

### Complicated Grieving (2006)—*cont'd*

**RELATED FACTORS**

- Emotional instability
- Lack of social support

**OUTCOME**

**Grief Resolution**

- Adjusts to loss

## Risk for Complicated Grieving (2006)

### DEFINITION

Presence of risk factors for a disorder that occurs after the death of a significant other, in which the experience of distress accompanying bereavement fails to follow normative expectations and manifests in functional impairment

### RISK FACTORS

- Death of a significant other
- Emotional instability
- Lack of social support

### OUTCOME

### Grief Resolution

- Adjusts to loss

## Dysfunctional Grieving  (1980, 1986, 2004)

### DEFINITION

Extended length or severity of grieving process (unresolved grieving) following an actual or perceived loss or change in pattern of relationships (includes people, possessions, job, status, home, ideals, and parts and processes of the body)

### DEFINING CHARACTERISTICS

#### Diagnostic Cues

♦ Verbal expression of distress/despair at a loss or denial of loss

and one of the following:

♦ Arrested grieving process before resolution
♦ Prolonged grieving beyond expected time for cultural group
♦ Emotional response more exaggerated than expected for cultural group (severity of reaction)

#### Supporting Cues

♦ Alterations in concentration and/or pursuits of tasks
♦ Expression of guilt, self criticism
♦ Expression of unresolved issues
♦ Sadness, anger, crying, labile affect
♦ Difficulty in expressing meaning of loss
♦ Alterations in activities of daily living: work, socialization, altered libido, change in eating habits, sleep–dream pattern
♦ Idealization of lost object
♦ Reliving past experiences, developmental regression
♦ Death anxiety

# ROLE–RELATIONSHIP PATTERN

## OUTCOME

### Grief Resolution

- Adjusts to actual loss
- Engages in life activities and roles

## ETIOLOGICAL OR RELATED FACTORS

- Loss or perceived loss or change (specify)
- Unavailable support systems

## HIGH-RISK POPULATIONS

- Preloss neuroticism
- Frequent major life events, changes
- History of psychiatric–mental health disorder
- Congenital anomaly
- Perinatal loss (later gestational age, length of life of infant, marital adjustment problems, past perinatal losses, absence of other living children)

### Chronic Sorrow (1998)

**DEFINITION**

Cyclical, recurring, and potentially progressive pattern of pervasive sadness, experienced in response to continual loss, throughout the trajectory of a chronic illness or disability

**DEFINING CHARACTERISTICS**

+ Describes differences or gap between current and former or desired situation
+ Expresses one or more of the following feelings that vary in intensity, are periodic, may progress and intensify over time, and may interfere with the client's ability to reach highest level of personal and social well-being
+ Periodic, recurrent feelings of sadness
+ Anger
+ Being misunderstood
+ Confusion
+ Depression; loneliness; emptiness
+ Disappointment; frustration
+ Fear
+ Guilt or self-blame
+ Helplessness; hopelessness; overwhelmed
+ Low self-esteem
+ Loss (recurring)

**OUTCOME**

**Psychosocial Adjustment: Life Change**

+ Adaptation to significant life change

# ROLE–RELATIONSHIP PATTERN

## ETIOLOGICAL OR RELATED FACTORS

- Chronic or life-threatening illness or disability (specify mental retardation, multiple sclerosis, infertility, cancer, Parkinson's disease, prematurity, spina bifida or other birth defects, chronic mental illness [e.g., schizophrenia, bipolar disorder, autism, dementia])
- Death of a loved one
- One or more trigger events (those circumstances, situations, and conditions that bring the disparity resulting from the loss experience clearly into focus or that exacerbate the experience of disparity)
- Crises in management of the illness
- Crises related to developmental stages and missed opportunities or milestones (that bring comparisons with developmental, social, or personal norms)
- Unending caregiving or other role changes that serve as a constant reminder of disparity between self and others

## HIGH-RISK POPULATIONS

- Individual or family caregiver experiencing continual loss throughout the trajectory of a chronic or life-threatening illness
- Bereaved individual in response to loss of a loved one
- Anatomical defect (e.g., cleft palate, altered neuromuscular visual system, auditory system, phonatory apparatus)

# ROLE–RELATIONSHIP PATTERN

## Ineffective Role Performance (Specify) (1978, 1996, 1998)

### DEFINITION

Change, conflict, denial of role responsibilities or inability to perform role responsibilities (specify type; this is a broad taxonomic category)

### DEFINING CHARACTERISTICS

- Denial of role
- Conflict in roles
- Change in self-perception of role
- Change in others' perception of role
- Change in physical capacity to resume role
- Lack of knowledge of role
- Change in usual patterns of responsibilities:
  - Role overload
  - Role dissatisfaction
  - Role confusion
  - Role strain
  - Role ambivalence

### OUTCOME

#### Role Performance

- Role behavior consistent with role expectation

## Unresolved Independence–Dependence Conflict

### DEFINITION

Need and desire to be dependent with a therapeutic, maturational, or social expectation to be independent; need and desire to be independent with a therapeutic, maturational, or social expectation to be dependent

### DEFINING CHARACTERISTICS

#### Diagnostic Cues

♦ Repeated verbal expressions of desire for independence (in situations that require some dependence: therapeutic, maturational, social)

or

♦ Repeated verbal expressions of desire for dependence (in situations that require independence; therapeutic, maturational, social)

and one or more of the following:

♦ Expression of anger
♦ Anxiety

### HIGH-RISK POPULATIONS

♦ Spinal cord injury
♦ Adolescents
♦ Bed rest confinement
♦ Degenerative chronic disease
♦ Physical activity restrictions

### OUTCOME

#### Conflict Resolution

♦ Acceptance of need for both independence and dependence

## Social Rejection* (1982)

### DEFINITION

Condition of aloneness experienced by the individual and perceived as imposed by others and as a negative or threatening state

### DEFINING CHARACTERISTICS

#### Diagnostic Cues

One or more of the following:

- Expresses feelings of aloneness imposed by others, feelings of rejection, feelings of difference from others
- Shows behavior unaccepted by dominant cultural group
- Expresses values acceptable to subculture but unacceptable to dominant cultural group
- Observed or expressed interests or activities inappropriate or not acceptable for the developmental age or stage

#### Supporting Cues

- Preoccupation with own thoughts, repetitive meaningless actions
- Perceived inability to meet expectations of others or insecurity in public
- Seeks to be alone or to exist in a subculture
- Perceived inadequacy of significant purpose in life or absence of purpose in life
- Sad, dull affect
- Uncommunicative, withdrawn, no eye contact
- Projects hostility in voice, behavior

*NANDA uses the term *Social Isolation* for this condition.

# ROLE–RELATIONSHIP PATTERN

## OUTCOME

### Social Involvement

- Interacts with others and participates in activities

## ETIOLOGICAL OR RELATED FACTORS

- Alteration in physical appearance or mental status
- Developmental delay (social skills)
- Immature interests
- Unacceptable social behavior or values
- Altered state of wellness
- Inability to engage in satisfying personal relationships

## HIGH-RISK POPULATIONS

- Mental disorders
- Observable disabilities, stigmata
- Retardation

## Social Isolation

### DEFINITION
Feelings of aloneness attributed to interpersonal interaction below level desired or required for personal integrity

### DEFINING CHARACTERISTICS
#### Diagnostic Cues
- Verbalization of isolation from others

and one or more of the following:
- Lack of contact with, or absence of, significant others
- Absent or limited contact with community
- Low contact with peers

#### Supporting Cues
- Apathy
- Seclusion

### OUTCOME
#### Social Involvement
- Interacts and participates in activities with others

### ETIOLOGICAL OR RELATED FACTORS
- Impaired mobility
- Therapeutic isolation
- Sociocultural dissonance
- Insufficient community resources
- Body image disturbance
- Fear (environmental hazards, violence)

### HIGH-RISK POPULATIONS
- Frail older persons
- Therapeutic isolation
- Disfigurement

ROLE–RELATIONSHIP PATTERN

## Impaired Social Interaction  (1986)

### DEFINITION
Insufficient or excessive quantity or ineffective quality of social exchange

### DEFINING CHARACTERISTICS
#### Diagnostic Cues
- Verbalized or observed discomfort in social situations (e.g., inability to receive or communicate a satisfying sense of belonging, caring, interest, or shared history)
- Observed use of unsuccessful social interaction behaviors

#### Supporting Cues
- Dysfunctional interaction with peers, family, others
- Family report of change of style or patterns of interaction

### OUTCOME
#### Social Involvement
- Productive social interactions with persons, groups, or organization

### ETIOLOGICAL OR RELATED FACTORS
- Knowledge or skill deficit (ways to enhance mutuality)
- Communication barriers
- Self-concept disturbance
- Absence of available significant others or peers (support system deficit)
- Limited physical mobility
- Therapeutic isolation
- Sociocultural dissonance
- Environmental barriers
- Altered thought processes
- Sensory deficit (vision, hearing)

357

## Developmental Delay: Social Skills (Specify)

### DEFINITION

Demonstrates deviations from age-group norms in acquisition of social skills

### DEFINING CHARACTERISTICS

#### Diagnostic Cues

+ Delay or difficulty in acquisition of social interaction skills typical of age group or developmental level
+ Dysfunctional interactions

### OUTCOME

#### Social Development

+ Acquisition of social skills is within age-group norm

### ETIOLOGICAL OR RELATED FACTORS

+ Environmental, stimulation, modeling deficiencies
+ Inconsistent responsiveness
+ Multiple caretakers, inadequate caretaking
+ Separation (from significant others)
+ Physical disability effects
+ Indifference
+ Self-esteem disturbance
+ Social isolation

### Relocation Stress Syndrome* (1992, 2000)

#### DEFINITION

Physiological and psychosocial disturbances resulting from transfer from one environment to another

#### DEFINING CHARACTERISTICS

#### Diagnostic Cues

- ♦ Change in environment or location
- ♦ Anxiety, apprehension, verbalization of being concerned or upset about transfer
- ♦ Reactive depression, sad affect, and/or increased confusion (older population)
- ♦ Expressions of loneliness
- ♦ Feeling of powerlessness or anger regarding move
- ♦ Sleep pattern disturbance and/or change in eating habits, gastrointestinal disturbances

#### Supporting Cues

- ♦ Moderate to high degree of environment change
- ♦ Unfavorable comparison of posttransfer with pretransfer staff
- ♦ Little or no preparation for impending move
- ♦ History of previous transfers (same or different type)
- ♦ Losses involved with decision to move
- ♦ Concurrent, recent, past losses
- ♦ Dependency
- ♦ Insecurity, lack of trust
- ♦ Support system deficit

*Continues*

---

*Generally, the probable cause (related or etiological factor) of a syndrome is contained in the name (e.g., relocation).

## Relocation Stress Syndrome (1992, 2000)—*cont'd*

+ Restlessness, vigilance, or withdrawal
+ Weight change
+ Impaired or decreased health status
  (psychosocial/physical)

**OUTCOME**

**Stress Level**

+ Low physical or mental tension resulting from factors
  that alter existing equilibrium

**HIGH-RISK POPULATIONS**

+ Lack of predeparture counseling/support
+ Language barrier
+ Isolation for family/friends
+ Unstable health status

## Risk for Relocation Stress Syndrome  (2000)

### DEFINITION

Risk for physiological and psychosocial disturbances resulting from transfer from one environment to another

### RISK FACTORS

- Moderate to high degree of environmental change (e.g., physical, ethnic, cultural)
- Temporary or permanent move
- Voluntary or involuntary move
- Lack of adequate support system/group
- Moderate mental competence (e.g., alert enough to experience changes)
- Unpredictability of experiences
- Decreased psychosocial or physical health status
- Lack of predeparture counseling
- Passive coping
- Past or current losses

### OUTCOME

### Stress Level

- Low physical or mental tension resulting from factors that may alter existing equilibrium

## Readiness for Enhanced Relationship (2008)

### DEFINITION

+ Pattern of mutual partnership sufficient to provide for each other's needs and can be strengthened

### DEFINING CHARACTERISTICS

+ Demonstrates mutual respect between partners
+ Expresses satisfaction with complementary relation between partners
+ Meets developmental goals appropriate for family life-cycle stage
+ Expresses desire to enhance communication between partners
+ Expresses satisfaction with sharing of information and ideas between partners
+ Expresses satisfaction with fulfilling partner's physical and emotional needs
+ Demonstrates well-balanced autonomy and collaboration between partners
+ Demonstrates mutual support in daily activities between partners
+ Identifies each other as a key person
+ Demonstrates understanding of partner's insufficient (physical, social, psychological) function

### OUTCOME

#### Relationships

+ Partnerships with others consistently provide for each other's needs

ROLE–RELATIONSHIP PATTERN

## Interrupted Family Processes (Specify) (1982, 1998)

### DEFINITION

Inability of family system (household members) to meet needs of members, carry out family functions, or maintain communications for mutual growth and maturation

### DEFINING CHARACTERISTICS

+ Inability of family members to relate to each other for mutual growth and maturation
+ Failure to send and receive clear messages
+ Poorly communicated family rules, rituals, symbols; unexamined myths
+ Unhealthy family decision-making processes
+ Inability of family members to express and accept wide range of feelings
+ Inability to accept and receive help
+ Does not demonstrate respect for individuality and autonomy of members
+ Rigidity in functions and roles
+ Fails to accomplish current (or past) family developmental tasks
+ Inappropriate (nonproductive) boundary maintenance
+ Inability to adapt to change
+ Inability to deal with traumatic or crisis experience constructively
+ Parents do not demonstrate respect for each other's views on child-rearing practices
+ Inappropriate (nonproductive) level and direction of energy
+ Inability to meet needs of members (physical, security, emotional, spiritual)
+ Family uninvolved in community activities

*Continues*

**Interrupted Family Processes (Specify) (1982, 1998)—*cont'd***

## OUTCOME

### Family Coping

+ Family actions manage stressors that tax family resources

### Family Functioning

+ Family system meets needs of its members during developmental transitions

## ETIOLOGICAL OR RELATED FACTORS

+ Situational crisis or transition (e.g., alcoholism of a member)
+ Developmental crisis or transition

## Dysfunctional Family Processes* (1994)

### DEFINITION

Psychosocial, spiritual, and physiological functions of family unit are chronically disorganized, leading to conflict, denial of problems, resistance to change, ineffective problem solving, and a series of self-perpetuating crises

### DEFINING CHARACTERISTICS
#### Roles and Relationships

- Deterioration in family relationships, disturbed family dynamics
- Ineffective spouse communication or marital problems
- Altered role function or disruption of family roles
- Inconsistent parenting or low perception of parental support
- Family denial
- Intimacy dysfunction, difficulty with intimate relationships
- Chronic family problems
- Closed communication systems

#### Behaviors

- Inappropriate expression of anger
- Loss of control of drinking
- Impaired communication
- Ineffective problem-solving skills
- Rationalization or denial of problems
- Enabling to maintain drinking
- Inability to meet emotional needs of family members
- Manipulation

*Continues*

*This diagnostic label was formerly Dysfunctional Family Processes: Alcoholism.

# ROLE–RELATIONSHIP PATTERN

## Dysfunctional Family Processes (1994)—*cont'd*

- Dependency
- Criticizing
- Alcohol abuse
- Broken promises
- Refusal to get help or inability to accept and receive help appropriately
- Blaming
- Inadequate understanding of alcoholism/drug abuse

### Feelings

- Decreased self-esteem, worthlessness, insecurity
- Anger or suppressed rage
- Frustration, powerlessness, hopelessness
- Anxiety, tension, distress
- Repressed emotions
- Responsibility for alcoholic's behavior
- Lingering resentment, hurt, shame, embarrassment
- Unhappiness, emotional isolation, loneliness, rejection
- Guilt
- Vulnerability
- Mistrust

### Supporting Cues

#### *Family Roles and Relationships*

- Triangulating family relationships
- Reduced ability of family members to relate to each other for mutual growth and maturation
- Lack of skills necessary for relationships
- Lack of cohesiveness, disrupted family rituals
- Family unable to meet security needs of its members, pattern of rejection

- Family does not demonstrate respect for individuality and autonomy of its members
- Economic problems, neglected obligations

### *Behaviors*

- Inability to meet spiritual needs of its members
- Inability to express or accept wide range of feelings
- Orientation toward tension relief rather than achievement of goals
- Family special occasions are alcohol centered
- Escalating conflict
- Lying
- Contradictory, paradoxical communication
- Lack of dealing with conflict
- Harsh self-judgment
- Isolation
- Substance abuse other than alcohol or nicotine addiction
- Difficulty having fun
- Self-blaming
- Unresolved grief
- Controlling communication or power struggles
- Inability to adapt to change
- Immaturity
- Stress-related physical illnesses
- Inability to deal with traumatic experiences constructively
- Seeking approval and affirmation
- Lack of reliability
- Disturbances in academic performance in children
- Disturbances in concentration
- Chaos
- Failure to accomplish current or past developmental tasks and difficulty with life-cycle transitions

*Continues*

## Dysfunctional Family Processes (1994)—*cont'd*

- ♦ Verbal abuse of spouse or parent
- ♦ Agitation
- ♦ Diminished physical contact

*Feelings*

- ♦ Being different from other people
- ♦ Depression
- ♦ Hostility
- ♦ Emotional control by others
- ♦ Confusion, lack of identity
- ♦ Dissatisfaction, moodiness
- ♦ Loss, abandonment
- ♦ Misunderstood
- ♦ Confused love and pity
- ♦ Failure; being unloved

## OUTCOME

### Family Coping

- ♦ Family manages stressors that tax family resources

### Family Functioning

- ♦ Family system meets needs of its members during developmental transitions

## ETIOLOGICAL OR RELATED FACTORS

- ♦ Abuse of alcohol, resistance to treatment
- ♦ Family history of alcoholism
- ♦ Inadequate coping skills
- ♦ Genetic predisposition, addictive personality
- ♦ Lack of problem-solving skills

**Readiness for Enhanced Family Processes (2002)**

## DEFINITION

Pattern of family functioning that is sufficient to support the well-being of family members and can be strengthened

## DEFINING CHARACTERISTICS

- Expresses desire to enhance family dynamics
- Family functioning meets physical, social, and psychological needs of family members
- Activities support the safety and growth of family members
- Communication is adequate
- Relationships are generally positive; interdependent with community; family tasks are accomplished
- Family roles are flexible and appropriate for developmental stages
- Respect for family members is evident
- Family adapts to change
- Boundaries of family members are maintained
- Energy level of family supports activities of daily living
- Family resilience is evident
- Balance exists between autonomy and cohesiveness

## OUTCOME

### Family Coping

- Family manages stressors that tax family resources

### Family Functioning

- Family system meets needs of its members during developmental transitions

## Impaired Parenting (Specify Impairment) (1978, 1998)

### DEFINITION

Inability of the primary caretaker to create an environment that promotes the optimal growth and development of the child (adjustment to parenting, in general, is a normal maturation process following the birth of a child)

### DEFINING CHARACTERISTICS

#### Parental

- Insecure attachment or lack of attachment to infant
- Maternal–child or parent–child interaction deficit
- Inability to recognize and act on infant cues
- Inconsistent or inappropriate caretaking skills
- Inconsistent behavior management
- Inconsistent care
- Inappropriate childcare arrangements
- Inflexibility to meet needs of child, situation
- Inadequate child health maintenance
- Inappropriate visual, tactile, auditory stimulation
- Negative statements about child
- Rejection of or hostility toward child
- Highly punitive
- Little cuddling
- Abandonment
- Child abuse
- Child neglect
- Preference for physical punishment
- Unrealistic expectations of child, self, partner
- Unsafe home environment
- Statements of inability to meet child's needs
- Verbalization that cannot control child
- Verbalizations of role inadequacy, frustration

# ROLE–RELATIONSHIP PATTERN

## Infant or Child

- Failure to thrive
- Lack of attachment (e.g., lack of separation anxiety)
- Poor cognitive development, poor academic performance
- Poor social competence
- Behavioral disorders, frequent illnesses, accidents
- Evidence of abuse
- Runaway

## OUTCOME

### Parenting Performance

- Parental actions provide a child with nurturing and constructive physical, emotional, and social environment

## ETIOLOGICAL OR RELATED FACTORS

### Physical Factors

- Sleep deprivation or disruption
- Infant or child handicapping condition or developmental delay

### Social Factors

- Not gender desired
- Parent–infant or parent–child prolonged separation
- Attention deficit–hyperactivity disorder
- Lack of fit between temperament of child and parental expectations
- Father of child not involved
- Marital conflict, declining satisfaction
- Lack of family cohesiveness
- Financial difficulties, poverty
- Unemployment or job problems

*Continues*

## Impaired Parenting (Specify Impairment) (1978, 1998)—*cont'd*

- Lack of resources or lack of access to resources (e.g., transportation)
- Legal difficulties
- Lack or poor parental role model
- Poor home environment
- Relocations
- Change in family unit
- Lack of value of parenthood
- Social isolation, social support network deficit
- Stress
- Role strain or overload
- Maladaptive coping strategies
- Poor problem-solving skills or communication skills
- Low self-esteem
- Inability to put child's needs before own

### Knowledge Factors

- Knowledge deficit (child development)
- Knowledge (parenting skills)
- Knowledge deficit (child health maintenance)
- Lack of cognitive readiness for parenthood
- Low cognitive functioning
- Poor communication skills

### HIGH-RISK POPULATIONS

- Disability
- Single parents
- Low socioeconomic class
- Low educational level or attainment
- History of being abused
- History of being abusive
- History of substance abuse, dependencies, mental illness

## ROLE–RELATIONSHIP PATTERN

- Unplanned or unwanted pregnancy
- Premature birth; difficult labor and delivery
- Young age, especially adolescent
- High number of closely spaced pregnancies
- Lack of or late prenatal care
- Multiple births
- Parent–infant separation at birth

## Risk for Impaired Parenting (Specify) (1978, 1998)

### DEFINITION
Risk for inability of primary caretaker to create, maintain, or regain an environment that promotes the optimal growth and development of the child (adjustment to parenting, in general, is a normal maturation process following the birth of a child)

### RISK FACTORS
#### Social Factors
+ Single parent
+ Father of child not involved
+ Lack of family cohesiveness
+ Poverty
+ Financial difficulties
+ Unemployment or job problems
+ Low socioeconomic class
+ Lack of resources and/or access to resources (e.g., transportation)
+ History of being abused
+ History of being abusive
+ Legal difficulties
+ Lack of or poor parental role model
+ Poor home environment
+ Relocation
+ Change in family unit
+ Lack of value of parenthood
+ Social isolation, social support network deficit
+ Role strain or overload
+ Maladaptive coping strategies or stress
+ Poor problem-solving or communication skills
+ Low self-esteem
+ Inability to put child's needs before own

- Unplanned or unwanted pregnancy
- Inadequate child care arrangements

### Knowledge Factors

- Unrealistic expectations of child
- Knowledge deficit (child development)
- Knowledge deficit (parenting skills)
- Knowledge deficit (child health maintenance)
- Lack of cognitive readiness for parenthood
- Low educational level or attainment, low cognitive functioning
- Inability to recognize and act on infant cues
- Preference for physical punishment

### Physical Factors

- Lack of or late prenatal care
- Young age, especially adolescent
- High number of closely spaced children
- Multiple birth
- Difficult labor and/or delivery
- Physical illness, disability
- Sleep deprivation or disruption

### Psychological Factors

- Marital conflict, declining satisfaction
- Separation from infant or child
- History of substance abuse or dependence
- History of mental illness
- Depression

### Infant/Child Factors

- Separation from parent at birth
- Prolonged separation from parent
- Premature birth

*Continues*

## Risk for Impaired Parenting (Specify) (1978, 1998)—cont'd

- Infant or child illness
- Handicapping condition or developmental delay
- Difficult temperament
- Lack of goodness of fit (temperament) with parental expectations
- Attention deficit–hyperactivity disorder
- Unplanned or unwanted child or not the gender desired
- Multiple birth
- Altered perceptual abilities

### OUTCOME

### Parenting Performance

- Parental actions provide child with nurturing and constructive physical, emotional, and social environment

## Parental Role Conflict  (1988)

### DEFINITION

Role confusion and conflict experienced by parent(s) in response to crisis

### DEFINING CHARACTERISTICS

#### Diagnostic Cues

One or more of the following:

+ Expresses concerns or feelings of inadequacy to provide for child's physical and emotional needs during hospitalization or in the home; is reluctant to participate in usual caretaking activities, even with encouragement and support
+ Expresses concerns about changes in parental role, family functioning, family communication, family health
+ Demonstrates disruption in caretaking routines
+ Expresses concern about perceived loss of control over decisions relating to child
+ Verbalizes or demonstrates feelings of guilt, anger, fear, anxiety, and/or frustrations about effect of a child's illness on family process (see Altered Family Process)

### OUTCOME

#### Parenting Performance

+ Parental actions provide child with nurturing and constructive physical, emotional, and social environment

*Continues*

## ETIOLOGICAL OR RELATED FACTORS

- Parent–child separation (because of chronic illness)
- Intimidation with invasive or restrictive modalities (e.g., isolation, intubation, specialized care centers, policies)
- Establishing home care of a child with special needs (e.g., apnea monitoring, postural drainage, hyperalimentation)
- Change in marital status
- Interruptions in family life caused by home-care regimen (treatments, caregivers, lack of respite)

## Weak Parent–Infant Attachment

### DEFINITION

Pattern of unreciprocal bonding relationship between parent and infant or primary caretaker and infant

### DEFINING CHARACTERISTICS

### Diagnostic Cues

*Infant*

- Infant does not respond to attempts to soothe or satisfy
- Inability of infant to give care-eliciting and/or behavioral cues
- Irritable infant or low responsiveness to parent

*Parent–Infant*

- Low reciprocal interaction pattern (e.g., minimal smiling, babbling response to touching, kissing)
- Absent or minimal eye contact

*Parent*

- Infrequent visitation of hospitalized infant (e.g., less than twice a week)
- Minimal smiling, close contact, enfolding, talking to baby
- Minimal touching, stroking, patting, rocking, holding, kissing of infant except when necessary to feed or change diapers
- Inappropriate or lack of parental response to infant cues (e.g., does not attempt comforting responses to crying or continues unsuccessful methods)
- Does not assume "en-face" position, eye-to-eye contact

*Continues*

## Weak Parent–Infant Attachment—*cont'd*

*Prenatal*

- Negative or ambivalent feelings regarding pregnancy continuing into third trimester

### Supporting Cues

- Few positive comments about infant, expressions of disappointment
- Bottle propped or tense posture during breastfeeding
- Prenatal history of ambivalence, negative or ambivalent feelings regarding pregnancy continuing into third trimester
- High-risk adolescent parent, physically or mentally ill parent
- Parental resentment of infant following maternal death or severe illness

### OUTCOME

### Parent–Infant Attachment

- Parent and infant behaviors demonstrate an enduring affectionate bond

### ETIOLOGICAL OR RELATED FACTORS

- Parental anxiety
- Fear (specify)
- Parent–infant separation
- Perceived low parenting competency (infant care)
- Low (infant) social responsiveness
- Support system deficit
- Family stress

## Risk for Impaired Attachment (1994)

### DEFINITION

Disruption of the interactive process between parent or significant other and infant that fosters the development of a protective and nurturing reciprocal relationship

### RISK FACTORS

- Inability of parents to meet personal needs
- Anxiety associated with the parent role
- Substance abuse
- Premature infant
- Ill infant or child who is unable to effectively initiate parental contact because of altered behavioral organization
- Parent–infant separation
- Physical barriers
- Lack of privacy

### OUTCOME

### Parent–Infant Attachment

- Parent and infant behaviors demonstrate an enduring affectionate bond

## Parent–Infant Separation

### DEFINITION

Presence of factors that prohibit interaction between infant and parent(s)

### DEFINING CHARACTERISTICS

#### Diagnostic Cues

- Verbalization by parent(s) indicating fear of interaction (e.g., fear that infant may die, fear of hurting infant)
- Infrequent contact with infant because of one or more of the following:
  - Inability of parent(s) to visit hospital regularly
  - Absent or limited opportunity for eye-to-eye contact between infant and parent(s)
  - Absent or limited opportunity for tactile interaction
  - Inability of infant to tolerate noise or touch
  - Lack of immediate access to infant

#### Supporting Cues

- Verbalization by parent(s) regarding inability to parent the infant because of separation or lack of knowledge about the infant
- Lack of immediate information regarding infant's condition

### OUTCOME

#### Parent–Infant Attachment

- Affectionate bond between infant and parent

## ETIOLOGICAL OR RELATED FACTORS

- ◆ Transportation difficulties for family to visit hospitalized infant
- ◆ Support system deficit (e.g., lack of care relief to enable visitation)

## HIGH-RISK POPULATIONS

- ◆ Prematurity
- ◆ Critical illness of infant or parent(s)
- ◆ Hospitalization of infant or parent(s)

## Readiness for Enhanced Parenting (2002)

### DEFINITION

Pattern of providing an environment for children or other dependent person(s) that is sufficient to nurture growth and development and can be strengthened

### DEFINING CHARACTERISTICS

+ Expresses desire to enhance parenting
+ Children and other dependent person(s) express satisfaction with home environment
+ Evidence of emotional and tacit support of children or dependent person(s)
+ Evidence of bonding/attachment
+ Meets physical and emotional needs of children/dependent person(s)
+ Exhibits realistic expectations of children/dependent person(s)

### OUTCOME

#### Parenting Performance

+ Parental actions provide child with a nurturing and constructive physical, emotional, and social environment

## Caregiver Role Strain  (1992, 1998, 2000)

### DEFINITION
Caregiver perceives difficulty in performing family caregiver role

### DEFINING CHARACTERISTICS
### Diagnostic Cues
Caregiver's report of one or more of the following:
- ♦ Inadequate resources to provide required care
- ♦ Difficulty completing required caregiving activities
- ♦ Worry about the care receiver (e.g., care receiver's health and emotional state, having to put the care receiver in an institution, and/or who will care for the care receiver if something should happen to the caregiver)
- ♦ Feeling that caregiving interferes with other important roles in caregiver's life
- ♦ Feeling of loss because the care receiver is "like a different person" compared with before caregiving began
- ♦ In the case of a child, feeling of loss that the care receiver was not the child the caregiver expected
- ♦ Family conflict around issues of providing care
- ♦ Stress or nervousness in caregiver's relationship with the care receiver
- ♦ Depression
- ♦ Dysfunctional change in caregiving activities
- ♦ Preoccupation with caregiving routine

*Continues*

### Caregiver Role Strain (1992, 1998, 2000)—*cont'd*

## Supporting Cues

*Caregiver Health Status*
**Physical Status**

- Gastrointestinal upset (mild stomach cramps, vomiting, diarrhea, recurrent gastric ulcer episodes)
- Weight change
- Rash
- Hypertension; cardiovascular disease
- Diabetes
- Fatigue, headaches

**Emotional Status**

- Impaired coping; lack of time to meet personal needs
- Disturbed sleep
- Anger, stress response
- Somatization
- Increased nervousness
- Emotionally labile
- Impatience, frustration

**Socioeconomic Status**

- Withdraws from social life
- Changes in leisure activities
- Refuses career advancement

## Caregiver–Care Receiver Relationship

- Grief/uncertainty regarding changed relationship with care receiver
- Difficulty watching care receiver go through the illness
- Family conflict
- Concerns about family members

# ROLE–RELATIONSHIP PATTERN

## OUTCOME
### Caregiver Performance: Direct Care

+ Provision by family care provider of appropriate personal and health care for a family member without stress

### Caregiver Performance: Indirect Care

+ Arrangement and oversight by family care provider of appropriate personal and health care for a family member

## ETIOLOGICAL OR RELATED FACTORS
### Pathophysiological/Physiological Factors

+ Illness severity, unpredictable course of illness, unstable health (care receiver)
+ Caregiver health impairment
+ Addiction or codependency
+ Discharge of family member with significant home care needs

### Developmental Factors

+ Caregiver not developmentally ready for caregiver role (e.g., young adult needing to provide care for a middle-aged parent)
+ Developmental delay or retardation (care receiver or caregiver)

### Psychosocial Factors

+ Psychological or cognitive problems (care receiver)
+ Deviant or bizarre behavior (care receiver)
+ Marginal family adaptation or dysfunction (before caregiving situation)
+ Marginal coping patterns (caregiver)

*Continues*

## Caregiver Role Strain  (1992, 1998, 2000)—*cont'd*

### Situational Factors

♦ Family or caregiver isolation
♦ Presence of abuse or violence
♦ Situational family stressors (e.g., significant loss, disaster or crisis, poverty or economic vulnerability, major life events: birth, death, hospitalization, leaving/returning home, marriage, divorce, employment changes, retirement)
♦ Duration of caregiving
♦ Inadequate physical environment for providing care (e.g., housing, transportation, community services, equipment)
♦ Lack of respite or recreation (caregiver)
♦ Inexperience with caregiving
♦ Competing role commitments (caregiver)
♦ Complexity or amount of caregiving tasks

### HIGH-RISK POPULATIONS

♦ Premature birth or congenital defect
♦ Significant home care needs
♦ Female caregiver; caregiver is spouse
♦ Family stress
♦ History of poor relationship (caregiver–care receiver)

## Risk for Caregiver Role Strain (1992)

### DEFINITION

Caregiver is vulnerable for perceived difficulty in performing the family caregiver role

### RISK FACTORS

#### Pathophysiological Risk Factors

- ♦ Illness severity, unpredictable course of illness, unstable health (care receiver)
- ♦ Caregiver health impairment
- ♦ Addiction or codependency
- ♦ Premature birth or congenital defect
- ♦ Discharge of family member with significant home care needs
- ♦ Caregiver is female
- ♦ Developmental risk factors
- ♦ Caregiver not developmentally ready for caregiver role (e.g., young adult needing to provide care for middle-aged parent)
- ♦ Developmental delay or retardation (care receiver or caregiver)

#### Psychological Risk Factors

- ♦ Psychological or cognitive problems (care receiver)
- ♦ Marginal family adaptation/dysfunction (before the caregiving situation)
- ♦ Marginal coping patterns (caregiver)
- ♦ History of poor relationship (caregiver–care receiver)
- ♦ Caregiver is spouse
- ♦ Deviant or bizarre behavior (care receiver)

*Continues*

## Risk for Caregiver Role Strain (1992)—*cont'd*

### Situational Risk Factors

+ Family or caregiver isolation
+ Presence of abuse or violence
+ Situational family stressors (specify; e.g., significant loss, disaster or crisis, poverty or economic vulnerability, major life events: birth, death, hospitalization, leaving or returning home, marriage, divorce, employment changes, retirement)
+ Duration of caregiving
+ Inadequate physical environment for providing care (e.g., housing, transportation, community services, equipment)
+ Lack of respite or recreation (caregiver)
+ Inexperience with caregiving
+ Competing role commitments (caregiver)
+ Complexity or amount of caregiving tasks

### OUTCOME

### Caregiver Performance: Direct Care

+ Provision by family care provider of appropriate personal and health care for a family member without stress

### Stress Level

+ Low physical or mental tension resulting from care-giving activities

# ROLE–RELATIONSHIP PATTERN

## Impaired Verbal Communication  (1983, 1996, 1998)

### DEFINITION
Reduced or absent ability to use language in human interaction

### DEFINING CHARACTERISTICS

#### Diagnostic Cues

- Difficulty expressing thoughts verbally (stuttering, slurring, trouble forming words or sentences) or unable to speak

and/or

- Reports difficulty understanding speech communications

#### Supporting Cues

- Inappropriate verbalization
- Dyspnea
- Unable to speak dominant language*

### OUTCOME

#### Communication

- Reception, interpretation, and expression of spoken, written and nonverbal messages

### ETIOLOGICAL OR RELATED FACTORS

- Psychological barrier (psychosis, lack of stimuli)
- Developmental or age related

### HIGH-RISK POPULATIONS

- Physical barrier (brain tumor, tracheostomy, intubation)
- Cultural difference*
- Anatomical defects (cleft palate)
- Decrease in circulation to brain

*May not indicate a nursing diagnosis—possibly a care delivery problem requiring a translator or establishing some means of nonverbal communication.

## Readiness for Enhanced Communication (2002)

### DEFINITION

Pattern of exchanging information and ideas with others that is sufficient for meeting needs and life goals and can be strengthened

### DEFINING CHARACTERISTICS

- Expresses willingness to enhance communication
- Able to speak or write a language
- Forms words, phrases, and language
- Expresses thoughts and feelings
- Uses and interprets nonverbal cues appropriately
- Expresses satisfaction with ability to share information and ideas with others

### OUTCOME

#### Communication

- Reception, interpretation, and expression of spoken, written and nonverbal messages

## ROLE–RELATIONSHIP PATTERN

### Developmental Delay: Communication Skills (Specify Type)

#### DEFINITION
Demonstrates deviations from age-group norms in development of communication skills (specify type of skill)

#### DEFINING CHARACTERISTICS
#### Diagnostic Cues

♦ Delay or difficulty in performing expressive, communication skills typical of age-group or developmental level (e.g., prelanguage vocalization, language skills, signs)

#### Supporting Cues

♦ Flat affect
♦ Listlessness
♦ Decreased responses

#### OUTCOME
#### Social Skills Development

♦ Development of communication skills meets norm for age group (specify type of skill)

#### ETIOLOGICAL OR RELATED FACTORS

♦ Environmental or stimulation deficiencies
♦ Inconsistent responsiveness; indifference
♦ Multiple caregivers, inadequate caregiving
♦ Separation (from significant others)
♦ Physical disability effects
♦ Prescribed dependence

## Risk for Other-Directed Violence (1980, 1996)

### DEFINITION

Behaviors in which an individual demonstrates that he/she can be physically, emotionally, and/or sexually harmful to others

### RISK FACTORS

- Body language (rigid posture, clenching of fists and jaw, hyperactivity, pacing, breathlessness, threatening stances)
- History of violence against others (e.g., hitting someone, kicking someone, spitting, scratching, biting, throwing objects at someone, rape or attempted rape, sexual molestation, urinating/defecating on a person)
- History of violence or threats (e.g., verbal threats against property or person, social threats, cursing, threatening notes or letters, threatening gestures, sexual threats)
- History of violent antisocial behavior (e.g., stealing, incessant borrowing, incessant demands for privileges, frequent interruption of meetings, refusal to eat, refusal to take medication, ignoring instructions)
- History of indirect violence (tearing off clothes, ripping objects off walls, writing on walls, urinating on floor, defecating on floor, stamping feet, having temper tantrums, running in corridors, yelling, throwing objects, breaking windows, slamming doors, making sexual advances)
- Other factors (neurological impairment, e.g., positive EEG, CAT, or MRI; head trauma, positive neurological findings, seizure disorders)
- Cognitive impairment (e.g., learning disabilities, attention deficit disorder, decreased intellectual functioning)

## ROLE–RELATIONSHIP PATTERN

- History of childhood abuse
- History of witnessing family violence
- Cruelty to animals, fire setting
- Prenatal and perinatal complications/abnormalities
- History of drug and/or alcohol abuse, pathological intoxication
- Psychotic symptomatology (e.g., auditory, visual, command hallucinations; paranoid delusions; loose, rambling or illogical thought processes)
- Motor vehicle offenses (e.g., frequent traffic violations, use of a motor vehicle to release anger)
- Suicidal behavior; impulsivity; availability or possession of weapon(s)

## OUTCOME

### Impulse Self-Control

- Self-restraint of compulsive or impulsive behavior involving others

**NOTES**

**NOTES**

**NOTES**

# Sexuality–
# Reproductive Pattern

## Ineffective Sexuality Patterns (1986, 2006)

### DEFINITION

Expression of concern regarding own sexuality

### DEFINING CHARACTERISTICS

- Altered achievement of perceived sex role
- Altered relationship with significant other
- Conflict involving values
- Reports difficulties in sexual behaviors or activities
- Reports limitations in sexual behaviors or activities
- Reports changes in sexual behaviors or activities

### OUTCOME

#### Sexual Identity

- Acknowledgment and acceptance of own sexuality

### ETIOLOGICAL OR RELATED FACTORS

- Ineffective or absent role model
- Knowledge or skill deficit (alternate responses to health-related transitions)
- Knowledge or skill deficit (altered body function or structure)
- Knowledge or skill deficit (illness or medical treatment)
- Lack of privacy
- Lack of significant other
- Ineffective or absent role models
- Conflicts with sexual orientation or variant preferences
- Fear (pregnancy)
- Fear (contacting a sexually transmitted disease)
- Impaired relationship with significant other

### Sexual Dysfunction (1980, 2006)

#### DEFINITION

Change in sexual function during the sexual response phases of desire, excitation, and/or orgasm which is viewed as unsatisfying, unrewarding, or inadequate

#### DEFINING CHARACTERISTICS

+ Verbalizations of problem in sexual relationships
    + Alterations in, or inability to achieve, sexual satisfaction
    + Alterations in achieving perceived sex role
    + Perceived alteration in sexual excitation and deficiency in desire
    + Inability to achieve desired sexual satisfaction
    + Seeks confirmation of desirability
    + Change of interest in self and others

#### OUTCOME

#### Sexual Functioning

+ Integrates physical, socioemotional, and intellectual aspects of sexual expression and performance

#### ETIOLOGICAL OR RELATED FACTORS

+ Ineffectual or absent role models
+ Physical abuse
+ Psychosocial abuse (e.g., harmful relationships)
+ Vulnerability
+ Misinformation or lack of knowledge
+ Lack of privacy

*Continues*

## Sexual Dysfunction (1980, 2006)—*cont'd*

- ♦ Lack of significant other
- ♦ Altered in relationship with significant other
- ♦ Values conflict

### HIGH-RISK POPULATIONS

- ♦ Altered body structure or function (pregnancy, recent childbirth, drugs, surgery, anomalies, disease process, trauma, radiation)

## Rape Trauma Syndrome* (1980, 1998)

### DEFINITION

Sustained maladaptive response to a forced, violent sexual penetration against the victim's will and consent

### DEFINING CHARACTERISTICS

#### Diagnostic Cues

*Acute Phase*

♦ Report of forced, violent, sexual penetration
and one or more of the following:
  ♦ Confusion
  ♦ Disorganization, mood swings
  ♦ Anxiety, agitation, aggression
  ♦ Nightmares or sleep disturbance
  ♦ Disassociative disorders, denial, depression
  ♦ Shock, anger, shame, guilt
  ♦ Humiliation, embarrassment, self-blame
  ♦ Feelings of vulnerability, hyperalertness
  ♦ Helplessness, powerlessness
  ♦ Inability to make decisions
  ♦ Dependence
  ♦ Fear of physical violence and death
  ♦ Muscle tension or spasms, gastrointestinal irritability
  ♦ Physical trauma (bruising, tissue irritation), genitourinary discomfort
  ♦ Paranoia
  ♦ Loss of self-esteem

*Continues*

---

*This syndrome includes the following three subcomponents: Rape Trauma, Compound Reaction, and Silent Reaction. In this text, each appears as a separate diagnosis.

**Rape Trauma Syndrome** (1980, 1998)—*cont'd*

*Long-Term*

♦ Changes in lifestyle, changes in residence
♦ Suicide attempts
♦ Phobias, substance abuse
♦ Sexual dysfunction
♦ Change in relationships
♦ Nightmares or sleep disturbance

## OUTCOME

### Abuse Recovery: Sexual

♦ Healing after physical/psychological injury

## Rape Trauma Syndrome: Compound Reaction (1980)

### DEFINITION

Forced, violent sexual penetration against the victim's will and consent. The trauma syndrome that develops from this attack or attempted attack includes an acute phase of disorganization of the victim's lifestyle and a long-term process of reorganization of lifestyle.

### DEFINING CHARACTERISTICS

See Defining Characteristics listed under Rape Trauma Syndrome

### Diagnostic Cues

- ♦ Reactivated symptoms of previous conditions (i.e., physical illness, psychiatric illness)
- ♦ Reliance on alcohol and/or drugs

### OUTCOME

### Abuse Recovery: Sexual

- ♦ Healing following physical/psychological injury

## Rape Trauma Syndrome: Silent Reaction (1980)

### DEFINITION

Presence of signs and symptoms but without victim's mentioning to anyone that rape has occurred

### DEFINING CHARACTERISTICS

See additional Defining Characteristics listed under Rape Trauma Syndrome

### Diagnostic Cues

+ No initial verbalization of the occurrence of rape
+ Abrupt changes in relationships with men
+ Increase in nightmares
+ Increasing anxiety during interview (blocking of associations, long periods of silence, minor stuttering, physical distress)
+ Marked changes in sexual behavior with opposite gender
+ Sudden onset of phobic reactions

### OUTCOME

### Abuse Recovery: Sexual

+ Healing after physical/psychological injury

# SEXUALITY–REPRODUCTIVE PATTERN

## Readiness for Enhanced Childbearing Process (2008)

### DEFINITION

A pattern of preparing for, maintaining, and strengthening a healthy pregnancy and childbirth process and care of newborn.*

### DEFINING CHARACTERISTICS

#### During Pregnancy

- Reports appropriate prenatal lifestyle (e.g., diet, elimination, sleep, bodily movement, exercise, personal hygiene)
- Reports appropriate physical preparations
- Reports managing unpleasant symptoms in pregnancy
- Demonstrates respect for unborn baby
- Reports a realistic birth plan
- Prepares necessary newborn care items
- Seeks necessary knowledge (e.g., of labor and delivery, newborn care)
- Reports availability of support systems
- Has regular prenatal health visits

#### During Labor and Delivery

- Reports lifestyle (e.g., diet, elimination, sleep, bodily movement, personal hygiene) that is appropriate for the stage of labor
- Responds appropriately to onset of labor
- Is proactive in labor and delivery
- Uses relaxation techniques appropriate for the stage of labor
- Demonstrates attachment behavior to the newborn baby
- Uses support systems appropriately

*Continues*

*The original Japanese term for "childbearing" is "Shussan Ikuji Koudou," which encompasses both childbirth and rearing of neonate. It is one of the main concepts of Japanese midwifery.

**Readiness for Enhanced Childbearing Process (2008)—*cont'd***

### After Birth*

- Demonstrates appropriate baby feeding techniques
- Demonstrates appropriate breast care
- Demonstrates attachment behavior to the baby
- Demonstrates basic baby care techniques
- Provides safe environment for the baby
- Reports appropriate postpartum lifestyle (e.g., diet, elimination, sleep, bodily movement, exercise, personal hygiene)
- Uses support systems appropriately

### OUTCOME

### Childbearing Process

- Prepares for, maintains, and strengthens pregnancy, childbirth process, and care of newborn

## Risk for Disturbed Maternal/Fetal Dyad  (2008)

### DEFINITION

Risk for disruption of symbiotic maternal/fetal dyad (as a result of co-morbid or pregnancy-related conditions)

### RISK FACTORS

- Complications of pregnancy (e.g., premature rupture of membranes, placenta previa or abruption, late prenatal care, multiple gestation)
- Compromised $O_2$ transport (e.g., anemia, cardiac disease, asthma, hypertension, seizures, premature labor, hemorrhage)
- Impaired glucose metabolism (e.g., diabetes, steroid use)
- Physical abuse
- Substance abuse (e.g., tobacco, alcohol, drugs)
- Treatment-related side effects (e.g., medications, surgery, chemotherapy)

### OUTCOME

- Maternal–fetal symbiosis during pregnancy

## NOTES

**NOTES**

## NOTES

# Coping–Stress

# Tolerance Pattern

## Ineffective Coping (Specify)* (1978, 1998)

### DEFINITION

Impairment of adaptive behaviors (valid appraisal, choice of response, and/or inability to use resources). Methods of handling stressful life situations are insufficient to prevent or control anxiety, fear, or anger. Specify stressor(s) (e.g., situational or maturational crises, uncertainty).

### DEFINING CHARACTERISTICS

#### Diagnostic Cues

- Reports presence of life stress or problems (specify)
- Reports feeling anxious, apprehensive, fearful, angry, and/or depressed
- Expresses inability to cope or ask for help
- Ineffective or inappropriate use of defense mechanisms (forms of coping that impede adaptive behavior, e.g., see avoidance coping, denial)

#### Supporting Cues

- Disturbance in pattern of tension release
- Disturbance in pattern of threat appraisal
- Inadequate resources (financial, etc.)
- Change in usual communication patterns
- Decrease in use of social support
- Poor concentration
- Lack of goal-directed behavior and resolution of problem (e.g., inability to attend to problem; difficulty organizing information)
- Inability to meet role expectations
- Inability to meet basic needs
- Destructive behavior toward self or others
- Sleep disturbance

*There may be gender differences in coping strategies.

- Fatigue
- Risk taking
- High illness rate
- Abuse of chemical agents
- High degree of perceived or actual threat

## OUTCOME

### Coping

- Employs personal actions to manage stressors that tax resources

### Psychosocial Adjustment: Life Change

- Adaptive psychosocial response to a significant life change

## ETIOLOGICAL OR RELATED FACTORS

- Inadequate problem solving
- Inadequate confidence in coping ability
- Inadequate perception of control
- Social support deficit or characteristics of relationships
- Inability to conserve adaptive energies

## HIGH-RISK POPULATIONS

- Inadequate opportunity to prepare for stressor

## COPING–STRESS TOLERANCE PATTERN

### Readiness for Enhanced Coping (2002)

**DEFINITION**

Pattern of cognitive and behavioral efforts to manage
demands that is sufficient for well-being and can be
strengthened

**DEFINING CHARACTERISTICS**

- Defines stressors as manageable
- Seeks social support
- Uses a broad range of problem- and emotion-oriented
  strategies
- Uses spiritual resources
- Acknowledges power
- Seeks knowledge of new strategies
- Is aware of possible environmental changes

**OUTCOME**

**Coping**

- Employs personal actions to manage stressors that tax
  resources

## Avoidance Coping*

### DEFINITION
Prolonged minimization or denial of information (facts, meanings, consequences) when a situation requires active coping

### DEFINING CHARACTERISTICS
#### Diagnostic Cues
+ Presence of perceived threat to health, self-image, values, lifestyle, or relationships
+ Minimizes, ignores, or forgets information following clear communication or observation
+ Mislabels events
+ Absence of problem solving, information seeking, incorporation of new information into future planning

#### Supporting Cues
+ Regressive dependency
+ Anxiety, depression, passivity, or anger

### OUTCOME
#### Coping
+ Employs personal actions to manage stressors that tax resources

### ETIOLOGICAL OR RELATED FACTORS
+ Perceived incompetency
+ Perceived powerlessness
+ Support system deficit
+ Independence–dependence conflict (adolescent)

---

*Avoidance is not to be confused with Hope or Adaptive Denial (see also Denial).

## Defensive Coping (1988)

### DEFINITION

Repeated projection of falsely positive self-evaluation based on a self-protective pattern that defends against underlying perceived threats to positive self-regard

### DEFINING CHARACTERISTICS

#### Diagnostic Cues

One or more of the following:

- Denial of obvious problems or weaknesses
- Projection of blame or responsibility
- Rationalization of failures
- Hypersensitivity to a slight or a criticism
- Grandiosity

#### Supporting Cues

- Superior attitude toward others
- Difficulty establishing or maintaining relationships
- Hostile laughter or ridicule of others
- Difficulty in reality testing of perceptions; reality distortion
- Lack of follow-through or participation in treatment or therapy

### OUTCOME

#### Coping

- Employs personal actions to manage stressors that threaten self esteem

### ETIOLOGICAL OR RELATED FACTORS

- Support system deficit
- Conflict between self perception and value system
- Fear of failure

# COPING–STRESS TOLERANCE PATTERN

- Fear of humiliation
- Fear of repercussions
- Lack of resilience
- Low level confidence in self and others
- Uncertainty
- Unrealistic self-expectations

## Ineffective Denial or Denial* (1988)

### DEFINITION

Conscious or unconscious attempt to reduce anxiety or fear by disavowing the knowledge or meaning of an event (to the detriment of health)

### DEFINING CHARACTERISTICS

#### Diagnostic Cues

- Unable to admit impact of disease or event on life pattern as manifested by one or more of the following:
  - Delays seeking or refuses health care to the detriment of health; does not admit fear of death or invalidism; displaces fear of impact of the condition; unrealistic plans
  - Selectively integrates information
  - Does not perceive danger or personal relevance of symptoms; minimizes symptoms or event

#### Supporting Cues

- Makes dismissive gestures or comments when speaking of distressing events
- Displaces source of symptoms to other organs

---

*It is unclear whether the adjective ineffective before the word denial relates to the diagnosis or its consequences. It is not consistent with definition and characteristics specified. Suggestion: use "Denial or Partial Denial," or see Avoidance Coping. Caution must be exercised in attempting to treat this condition (helping the patient to recognize fully a threat or danger) during a crisis situation (e.g., surgery, infarct).

- ◆ Inconsistent expression of fear or anxiety
- ◆ Displays inappropriate affect
- ◆ Uses home remedies (e.g., self-treatment) to relieve symptoms

## OUTCOME

### Anxiety Level

- ◆ Absence of apprehension, tension, or uneasiness
- ◆ Discusses distressing events/impact of disease

## COPING–STRESS TOLERANCE PATTERN

### Impaired Resilience (Individual) (2008)

**DEFINITION**

Decrease ability to sustain a pattern of positive responses to an adverse situation or crisis

**DEFINING CHARACTERISTICS**

- Decreased interest in academic activities
- Decreased interest in vocational activities
- Depression
- Guilt
- Isolation
- Low self-esteem
- Lower perceived health status
- Renewed elevation of distress
- Shame
- Social isolation
- Using maladaptive coping skills (e.g., drug use, violence)

**OUTCOME**

- Positive coping responses to adverse situations or crisis

**ETIOLOGICAL OR RELATED FACTORS**

- Demographics that increase chance of maladjustment
- Drug use
- Inconsistent parenting
- Low intelligence
- Parental mental illness
- Poor impulse control
- Poverty
- Psychological disorders

# COPING–STRESS TOLERANCE PATTERN

- Vulnerability factors which encompass indices that exacerbate the negative effects of the risk condition
- Violence
- Violence in neighborhood

## HIGH-RISK POPULATIONS

- Minority status
- Large family size
- Gender
- Low maternal education

## Risk for Compromised Resilience (2008)

**DEFINITION**

At risk for decreased ability to sustain a pattern of positive responses to an adverse situation or crisis

**RISK FACTORS**

- Chronicity of existing crises
- Multiple coexisting adverse situations
- Presence of an additional new crisis (e.g., unplanned pregnancy, death of a spouse, loss of job, illness, loss of housing, death of family member)

**OUTCOME**

- Consistently uses positive coping responses to adverse situations or crisis

## Readiness for Enhanced Resilience* (2008)

### DEFINITION

A pattern of positive responses to an adverse situation or crisis that can be strengthened to optimize human potential

### DEFINING CHARACTERISTICS

- Access to resources
- Demonstrates positive outlook
- Effective use of conflict management strategies
- Enhances personal coping skills
- Expressed desire to enhance resilience
- Identifies available resources
- Identifies support systems
- Increases positive relationships with others
- Involvement in activities
- Makes progress toward goals
- Presence of a crisis
- Safe environment is maintained
- Sets goals
- Takes responsibilities for actions
- Use of effective communication skills
- Verbalizes an enhanced sense of control
- Verbalizes self-esteem

### OUTCOME

### Coping

- Positive coping responses to adverse situations or crisis

*NANDA-I lists related factors for this diagnosis (see Impaired Resilience for these).

## Compromised Family Coping (1980, 1996)

### DEFINITION

Usually supportive primary person (family member or close friend) providing insufficient, ineffective, or compromised support, comfort, assistance, or encouragement, which may be needed by client to manage or master adaptive tasks related to health challenge

### DEFINING CHARACTERISTICS

#### Diagnostic Cues

- ◆ Client or another person expresses concern or complaint about significant other's response to client's health problem

and one or more of the following:

- ◆ Significant person displays protective behavior disproportionate (too little or too much) to client's abilities or need for autonomy
- ◆ Significant person describes preoccupation with personal reactions (e.g., fear, guilt, anticipatory grief, anxiety) to client's illness, disability, or other situational or developmental crises
- ◆ Significant person describes or confirms inadequate understanding of knowledge base that interferes with effective assistive or supportive behaviors (specify)
- ◆ Significant person withdraws or enters into limited or temporary personal communication with client at time of need
- ◆ Significant person attempts assistive or supportive behaviors with less than satisfactory results

## COPING–STRESS TOLERANCE PATTERN

### OUTCOME

### Caregiver Performance: Direct Care/Indirect Care

+ Family care provider provides appropriate health and personal care for a family member

### ETIOLOGICAL OR RELATED FACTORS

+ Knowledge deficit (specify area)
+ Emotional conflicts (specify)
+ Exhaustion of supportive capacity (see Caregiver Role Strain)
+ Role changes (family)
+ Temporary family disorganization
+ Developmental or situational crises (specify)

### HIGH-RISK POPULATIONS

+ 24-hour home care
+ Home care with periodic health crises
+ History of family life stresses

## Disabled Family Coping (1980, 1996)

### DEFINITION

Behavior of significant person (family member or primary person) disables own capacities and client's capacities to effectively address tasks essential to either person's adaptation to the health challenge

### DEFINING CHARACTERISTICS

#### Diagnostic Cues

+ Neglectful care of client in regard to basic human needs and/or illness treatment

and one or more of the following:

+ Distortion of reality regarding client's health problem, including extreme denial about existence or severity (see also Denial)
+ Intolerance
+ Rejection
+ Abandonment
+ Desertion
+ Carrying on usual routines, disregarding client's needs
+ Psychosomaticism
+ Taking on illness signs of the client
+ Decisions and actions by family that are detrimental to economic or social well-being
+ Agitation, depression, aggression, hostility
+ Impaired restructuring of a meaningful life for self, impaired individuation, prolonged overconcern for client
+ Neglectful relationships with other family members
+ Client's development of helpless, inactive dependence

# COPING–STRESS TOLERANCE PATTERN

## OUTCOME

### Caregiver Performance: Direct Care/Indirect Care

- Family care provider provides appropriate health and personal care for a family member

## ETIOLOGICAL OR RELATED FACTORS

- Chronically unexpressed guilt, anxiety, hostility by significant other
- Dissonant discrepancy of coping styles (for dealing with adaptive tasks by the significant person and client or among significant people)
- Highly ambivalent family relationships
- Arbitrary handling of family's resistance to treatment (tends to solidify defensiveness as it fails to deal adequately with underlying anxiety)

## HIGH-RISK POPULATIONS

- 24-hour home care
- History of family life stresses
- Home care with periodic health crises

## Readiness for Enhanced Family Coping (1980)

### DEFINITION

Effective management of adaptive tasks involved with the client's health challenge by family member, who now exhibits desire and readiness for enhanced health and growth in regard to self and in relation to the client

### DEFINING CHARACTERISTICS

+ Family member moves in direction of health-promoting and enriching lifestyle that supports and monitors maturational processes, audits and negotiates treatment programs and generally chooses experiences that optimize wellness
+ Individual expresses interest in making contact on a one-to-one basis or on a mutual-aid group basis with another person who has experienced a similar situation
+ Family member attempts to describe growth impact of crisis on own values, priorities, goals, or relationships

### OUTCOME

#### Caregiver Performance: Direct Care/Indirect Care

+ Family care provider consistently provides appropriate health and personal care for a family member

## Ineffective Community Coping (1994, 1998)

### DEFINITION

Pattern of community activities for problem solving that is unsatisfactory for meeting the demands or needs of the community

### DEFINING CHARACTERISTICS

- Community does not meet its own expectations
- Deficits in community participation
- Excessive community conflicts
- Expressed vulnerability
- Expressed community powerlessness
- High illness rates
- Stressors perceived as excessive
- Increased social problems (e.g., homicides, vandalism, arson, terrorism, robbery, infanticide, abuse, divorce, unemployment, poverty, militancy, mental illness)

### OUTCOME

#### Community Competence

- Community collectively problem solves to achieve community goals

### ETIOLOGICAL OR RELATED FACTORS

#### Community Social Support Deficit

- Inadequate resources for problem solving
- Ineffective or nonexistent community systems (e.g., lack of emergency medical system, transportation systems, disaster planning systems)

### HIGH-RISK POPULATIONS

- Natural or manmade disasters

431

## Readiness for Enhanced Community Coping (1994)

### DEFINITION

Pattern of community activities for adaptation and problem solving that is satisfactory for meeting the demands or needs of the community but can be improved for management of current and future problems or stressors

### DEFINING CHARACTERISTICS

- ◆ Deficits in one or more characteristics that indicate effective coping
- ◆ Active planning by community for predicted stressors
- ◆ Active problem solving by community when faced with issues
- ◆ Agreement that community is responsible for stress management
- ◆ Positive communication among community members
- ◆ Positive communication between community and/or aggregates and larger community
- ◆ Programs available for recreation and relaxation
- ◆ Resources sufficient for managing stressors

### OUTCOME

#### Community Competence

- ◆ Community collectively problem solves to achieve community goals

### ETIOLOGICAL OR RELATED FACTORS

- ◆ Social supports available
- ◆ Resources available for problem solving
- ◆ Community has a sense of power to manage stressors

## Posttrauma Syndrome  (1986, 1998)

### DEFINITION

Sustained, maladaptive response to a traumatic overwhelming event

### DEFINING CHARACTERISTICS

### Reaction

- ♦ Intrusive thoughts
- ♦ Detachment
- ♦ Psychogenic amnesia
- ♦ Hypervigilance
- ♦ Substance abuse
- ♦ Compulsive behavior
- ♦ Avoidance, alienation
- ♦ Shame, guilt
- ♦ Grief, hopelessness
- ♦ Denial, repression

### Emotional/Cognitive

- ♦ Sadness, depression
- ♦ Anxiety, fear
- ♦ Horror
- ♦ Anger, rage, aggression
- ♦ Irritability
- ♦ Panic attacks
- ♦ Difficulty in concentrating
- ♦ Flashbacks, exaggerated startle response

*Continues*

## Posttrauma Syndrome (1986, 1998)—*cont'd*

### Physical

- Gastric irritability
- Neurosensory irritability, palpitations
- Headaches
- Enuresis (in children)

### Sleep

- Intrusive dreams
- Nightmares

## OUTCOME

### Anxiety Level

- Absence of apprehension, tension, or uneasiness

## HIGH-RISK POPULATIONS

- Events outside the range of usual human experience
- Natural or manmade disasters
- Witnessing mutilation, violent death, or other horrors
- Sudden destruction of one's home or community
- Tragic occurrence involving multiple deaths
- War or military combat
- Serious threat or injury to self or loved ones
- Held prisoner of war or criminal victimization (torture)
- Serious industrial and motor vehicle accidents
- Physical and psychological abuse

## Risk for Posttrauma Syndrome (1998)

### DEFINITION
Risk for sustained maladaptive response to a traumatic over-whelming event

### RISK FACTORS
- Nonsupportive environment
- Inadequate social support
- Survivor's role in the event
- Exaggerated sense of responsibility
- Perception of event
- Duration of event
- Occupation (police, fire, rescue, corrections, emergency room staff, mental health provider)
- Displacement from home
- Diminished ego strength

### OUTCOME
#### Stress Level
- Absence of physical or mental tension resulting from factors that alter an existing equilibrium

## Support System Deficit*

### DEFINITION

Insufficient emotional and/or instrumental help from others

### DEFINING CHARACTERISTICS

One or more of the following:

- ♦ Lack of one or more persons who communicates positive regard about personal worth and competence
- ♦ Insufficient or absent social network to provide instrumental assistance (e.g., transportation, household tasks)
- ♦ Lack or unavailability of a confidant

### Supporting Cues

- ♦ Absence of visitors
- ♦ Reports feeling anxious or apprehensive
- ♦ Reports feeling depressed
- ♦ Disorganized behavior
- ♦ Reports somatic complaints
- ♦ Irritable or hostile

### OUTCOME

### Supportive Environment

- ♦ Experiences positive regard and instrumental assistance from others when appropriate

### HIGH-RISK POPULATIONS

- ♦ Older without family and experiencing death of friends
- ♦ Small or absent social network

---

*This condition is frequently a focus for intervention (i.e., etiological/related factors).

436

### Risk for Suicide (2000)

**DEFINITION**

Presence of risk factors for self-inflicted, life-threatening injury

**RISK FACTORS**

**Behavioral**

- History of prior suicide attempt
- Impulsiveness
- Buying a gun
- Stockpiling medicines
- Making or changing a will
- Giving away possessions
- Sudden euphoric recovery from major depression
- Marked changes in behavior, attitude, school performance

**Verbal**

- Threats of killing oneself
- States desire to die/"end it all"

**Situational**

- Living alone
- Retired
- Relocation, institutionalization
- Economic instability
- Loss of autonomy/independence
- Presence of gun in the home
- Adolescents living in nontraditional settings (e.g., juvenile detention center, prison, half-way house, group home)

*Continues*

## Risk for Suicide (2000)—*cont'd*

### Psychological

- Family history of suicide
- Alcohol and substance use/abuse
- Psychiatric illness/disorder (e.g., depression, schizophrenia, bipolar disorder)
- Abuse in childhood
- Guilt
- Gay or lesbian youth

### Demographic

- Age: Older person, young adult, adolescents
- Race: Caucasian, Native American
- Gender: Male
- Marital Status: Divorced, widowed

### Physical

- Physical illness, terminal illness
- Chronic pain

### Social

- Loss of important relationship
- Disrupted family life
- Grief, bereavement
- Support system deficit
- Loneliness
- Hopelessness, helplessness
- Social isolation
- Legal or disciplinary problem
- Cluster suicides

## OUTCOME

### Risk Control

- Employs personal actions to prevent, eliminate, or reduce modifiable threat

### Will to Live

- Desires, and uses determination and effort, to survive life challenges

### Stress Overload (2006)

## DEFINITION

Excessive amounts and types of demands that require action

## DEFINING CHARACTERISTICS

### Diagnostic Cues

- Intense, repeated or co-existing stressors (e.g., family violence, chronic illness, terminal illness, environmental threats/demands, physical threats/demands, social threats/demands)
- Reports situational stress as excessive (e.g., rates stress level as seven or above on a 10-point scale)
- Reports negative impact from stress (e.g., physical symptoms, psychological distress, feeling of "being sick" or of "going to get sick")
- Expresses feelings of tension, pressure, and/or difficulty in functioning

### Supporting Cues

- Expresses feelings of anger and/or impatience
- Expresses problems with decision making

## OUTCOME

### Stress Level

- Reports less demands producing tension
- Expresses feeling of relaxation

## ETIOLOGICAL OR RELATED FACTORS

- Inadequate resources (e.g., financial, social, education/knowledge level)

## DEFINITION

Deliberate self-injurious behavior causing tissue damage with the intent of causing nonfatal injury to attain relief of tension

## DEFINING CHARACTERISTICS

- History of self-injurious behavior
- Cuts/scratches on body
- Picking at wounds
- Self-inflicted burns (e.g., eraser, cigarette)
- Ingestion/inhalation of harmful substances/objects
- Biting; abrading; severing; hitting; constricting a body part
- Insertion of object(s) into body orifice(s)

## OUTCOME

### Self-Mutilation Restraint

- Employs personal actions to refrain from intentional self-inflicted injury (nonlethal)

## ETIOLOGICAL OR RELATED FACTORS

- Adolescence; fluctuating emotions
- Childhood illness or surgery, foster, group, or institutional care
- Incarceration
- Isolation from peers
- Perfectionism
- Low or unstable body image
- Command hallucinations; sexual identity crisis
- History of inability to plan solutions or see long-term consequences

*Continues*

## Self-Mutilation  (2000)—*cont'd*

- Dysfunctional family (violence between parental figures; family alcoholism/divorce/history of self-destructive behavior)
- Use of manipulation to obtain nurturing relationship with others
- Chaotic/disturbed interpersonal relationships
- Childhood sexual abuse; substance abuse; eating disorder
- Emotionally disturbed and/or battered children
- Feels threatened with actual or potential loss of significant relationship (e.g., loss of parent or parental relationships)
- Experiences dissociation or depersonalization; character disorders; borderline personality disorders
- Feelings of depression, rejection, self hatred, separation anxiety, guilt and depersonalization

### HIGH-RISK POPULATIONS

- Borderline personality disorder, especially females 16 to 25 years of age
- Psychotic state; frequently males in young adulthood
- Emotionally disturbed and/or battered children
- Mentally retarded and autistic children
- History of self-injury or history of physical, emotional, or sexual abuse

## Risk for Self-Mutilation (1992, 2000)

### DEFINITION

Presence of risk factors for deliberate self-injurious behavior causing tissue damage with the intent of causing nonfatal injury to attain relief of tension

### RISK FACTORS

- Inability to cope with increased psychological or physiological tension in a healthy manner
- Experiences mounting tension that is intolerable
- Impulsivity
- Inability to express tension verbally; experiences irresistible urge to cut/damage self
- Needs quick reduction of stress
- Rationalizations or rejections of positive feedback
- Feelings of depression, rejection, self-hatred, separation anxiety, guilt, depersonalization
- Peers who self mutilate
- Adolescence; fluctuating emotions
- Childhood illness or surgery, foster, group, or institutional care
- Incarceration
- Isolation from peers
- Perfectionism
- Low or unstable body image
- Command hallucinations; sexual identity crisis
- History of inability to plan solutions or see long-term consequences
- Need for sensory stimuli
- Parental emotional deprivation

*Continues*

## Risk for Self-Mutilation (1992, 2000)—*cont'd*

- Dysfunctional family (violence between parental figures; family alcoholism/divorce/history of self-destructive behavior)
- Use of manipulation to obtain nurturing relationship with others
- Chaotic/disturbed interpersonal relationships
- Childhood sexual abuse; substance abuse; eating disorder
- Emotionally disturbed and/or battered children
- Feels threatened with actual or potential loss of significant relationship
- Loss of parent or parental relationships
- Experiences dissociation or depersonalization; character disorders; borderline personality disorders
- Loss of control over problem-solving situations
- Developmental delay or autism
- History of self-injurious behavior
- Feelings of depression, rejection, self hatred, separation anxiety, guilt and depersonalization

## OUTCOME

### Self-Mutilation Restraint

- Employs personal actions to refrain from intentional self-inflicted injury (nonlethal)

**NOTES**

## NOTES

# Value–Belief Pattern

## Moral Distress  (2007)

### DEFINITION

Anguish in response to the inability to carry out one's chosen ethical/moral decision/action

### DEFINING CHARACTERISTICS

- Expresses anguish (e.g., powerlessness, guilt, frustration, anxiety, self-doubt, fear) over difficulty acting on one's moral choice

### RELATED FACTORS

- Conflict among decision makers
- Conflicting information guiding ethical decision making
- Conflicting information guiding moral decision making
- Cultural conflicts
- End-of-life decisions
- Loss of autonomy
- Physical distance of decision maker
- Time constraints for decision making
- Treatment decisions

### OUTCOME

**Distress Resolution**

- Resolves conflicting situation

## Spiritual Distress  (1978, 2002)

### DEFINITION

Impaired ability to experience and integrate meaning and purpose in life through a connectedness with self, others, art, music, literature, or a power greater than oneself

### DEFINING CHARACTERISTICS

#### Connections to Self

- ♦ Expresses one or more of the following: lack of hope, meaning and purpose in life, peace/serenity, acceptance, love, forgiveness of self, courage
- ♦ Anger
- ♦ Guilt
- ♦ Poor coping

#### Connections with Others

- ♦ Refuses interactions with spiritual leaders
- ♦ Refuses interactions with friends, family
- ♦ Verbalizes being separated from support system
- ♦ Expresses alienation

#### Connection with Art, Music Literature, Nature

- ♦ Inability to express previous state of creativity (singing/listening to music/writing)
- ♦ No interest in nature
- ♦ No interest in reading spiritual literature

#### Connections with Power Greater than Self

- ♦ Inability to pray
- ♦ Inability to participate in religious activities
- ♦ Expresses being abandoned by or having anger toward God

*Continues*

## Spiritual Distress  (1978, 2002)—*cont'd*

+ Inability to experience transcendence
+ Request to see a religious leader
+ Sudden changes in spiritual practices
+ Inability to be introspective/inward turning
+ Expresses being without hope, suffering

## OUTCOME

### Spiritual Health

+ Connectedness with self, others, higher power, all life, nature, and the universe that transcends and empowers the self

## ETIOLOGICAL OR RELATED FACTORS

+ Self-alienation
+ Loneliness
+ Social alienation
+ Anxiety
+ Sociocultural deprivation
+ Death and dying of self or others
+ Pain
+ Life change
+ Chronic illness of self or others

## Risk for Spiritual Distress  (1998, 2004)

### DEFINITION
Presence of risk factors for an impaired ability to experience and integrate meaning and purpose in life through connectedness with self, other persons, art, music, literature, nature, and/or a power greater than oneself

### RISK FACTORS
#### Physical

- Physical illness
- Substance abuse/excessive drinking
- Chronic illness

#### Psychosocial

- Low self-esteem
- Depression
- Stress/anxiety
- Poor relationships
- Separated from support systems
- Blocks to experiencing love
- Inability to forgive
- Loss
- Racial/cultural conflict
- Change in religious rituals or spiritual practices

#### Developmental

- Life change

#### Environmental

- Environmental changes
- Natural disasters

*Continues*

## Risk for Spiritual Distress (1998, 2004)—*cont'd*

**OUTCOME**

### Spiritual Health

- Connectedness with self, others, higher power, all life, nature, and the universe that transcends and empowers the self

## Readiness for Enhanced Spiritual Well-Being (1994, 2002)

### DEFINITION

Ability to experience and integrate meaning and purpose in life through connectedness with self, others, art, music, literature, nature, or a power greater than oneself

### DEFINING CHARACTERISTICS

#### Connections to Self

- Desire for enhanced hope, meaning and purpose in life, peace, serenity, acceptance, surrender, love, forgiveness of self, satisfying philosophy of life, joy, courage
- Heightened coping
- Meditation

#### Connections with Others

- Provides service to others
- Requests interactions with spiritual leaders
- Requests forgiveness of others
- Requests interactions with friends, family

#### Connections with Art, Music, Literature, Nature

- Displays creative energy (writing, poetry)
- Sings/listens to music
- Reads spiritual literature
- Spends time outdoors

*Continues*

**Readiness for Enhanced Spiritual Well-Being (1994, 2002)—*cont'd***

## Connections with Power Greater than Self

- Prays
- Reports mystical experience
- Participates in religious activities
- Expresses reverence, awe

## OUTCOME

## Spiritual Health

- Connectedness with self, others, higher power, all life, nature, and the universe that transcends and empowers the self

## Impaired Religiosity (2004)

### DEFINITION

Impaired ability to rely on beliefs and/or participate in rituals of a particular faith tradition

### DEFINING CHARACTERISTICS

- ◆ Demonstrates or expresses difficulty adhering to prescribed religious beliefs and rituals (e.g., religious ceremonies, dietary regulations, clothing, prayer, worship/religious services, private religious behaviors/ reading religious materials/media, holiday observances, meeting with religious leaders)
- ◆ Expresses need to reconnect with previous belief patterns and customs
- ◆ Expresses emotional distress because of separation from faith community
- ◆ Questions religious belief patterns and customs*
- ◆ Expresses emotional distress regarding religious beliefs and/or religious social network*

### OUTCOME

#### Religious Support

- ◆ Finds support in personal beliefs and/or participates in rituals of a particular faith tradition

### ETIOLOGICAL OR RELATED FACTORS

- ◆ Pain/suffering
- ◆ Ineffective coping (e.g., with disease)
- ◆ Deficient support system
- ◆ Lack of security

*Continues*

*See Spiritual Distress, p. 429.

## Impaired Religiosity (2004)—*cont'd*

- ◆ Anxiety
- ◆ Fear of death
- ◆ Cultural barriers (to practicing religion)
- ◆ Environmental barriers (to practicing religion)
- ◆ Lack of social integration
- ◆ Lack of social/cultural interaction
- ◆ Spiritual distress (spiritual crisis)
- ◆ Use of religion to manipulate

### HIGH-RISK POPULATIONS

- ◆ End-stage life crises
- ◆ Aging
- ◆ Sickness/illness
- ◆ Personal disaster/crisis
- ◆ Life transitions

## Risk for Impaired Religiosity (2004)

### DEFINITION

Presence of risk factors for impaired ability to rely on religious beliefs and/or participate in rituals of a particular faith tradition

### RISK FACTORS

- Illness/hospitalization
- Pain
- Suffering
- Ineffective coping
- Deficient support system
- Depression
- Lack of security
- Lack of social interaction
- Cultural barriers to practicing religion
- Environmental barriers to practicing religion
- Social isolation
- Lack of transportation
- Life transitions

### OUTCOME

#### Religious Support

- Finds support in personal beliefs and/or participates in rituals of a particular faith tradition

# VALUE–BELIEF PATTERN

## Readiness for Enhanced Religiosity (2004)

### DEFINITION

Desire/ability to increase reliance on religious beliefs and/or participate in rituals of a particular faith community

### DEFINING CHARACTERISTICS

* Expresses desire to strengthen religious belief patterns and customs that have provided comfort/religion in the past
* Request for assistance to increase participation in prescribed religious beliefs through religious ceremonies, dietary regulations/rituals, clothing, prayer, worship/religious services, private religious behaviors/reading religious materials/media, holiday observances
* Requests assistance expanding religious options
* Requests meeting with religious leaders/facilitators
* Requests forgiveness, reconciliation
* Requests religious material and/or experiences
* Questions or rejects belief patterns and customs that are harmful

### OUTCOME

### Religious Support

* Finds support in personal beliefs and/or participates in rituals of a particular faith tradition

**NOTES**

**NOTES**

# Glossary

# GLOSSARY

**Approved nursing diagnoses**  Health-related conditions submitted by nurses that have been reviewed and accepted as nursing diagnoses by NANDA International; classes or categories of health problems in a nursing diagnostic classification system.

**Assessment**  The collection and interpretation of clinical data; a health-status evaluation done by a health professional.

**Defining characteristic**  An observable sign, verbal report, or contextual attribute that increases the probability of a diagnosis; serves as a cue or indicator of a diagnosis; a sign or symptom; a historical or current indicator of client-environment interaction; a human response.

**Diagnostic cue**  An observable sign, verbal report, or contextual attribute that serves as a critical indicator of a health problem; a specific criterion that strongly influences the probability of a diagnosis; a sign or symptom that is usually present when a specific diagnosis is present; a defining characteristic.

**Documentation**  Recording of observations, judgments, actions, test results, events, and plans related to the health or health care of an individual, family, or community; may be entries in a computer or on paper documents.

**Etiological factors**  Probable causes of a health problem; usually research-based, causal relationships.

**Functional health pattern**  A configuration (interrelated information) of health-related behaviors that occurs sequentially across time; sequences of health-related behaviors; a specific division in a typology.

**High-risk population**  Individuals, families, or groups that have a greater than average risk for a condition described by a nursing diagnosis.

**North American Nursing Diagnosis Association (name changed to NANDA International in 2004)**  An organization of American and Canadian nurses and nurses from other countries dedicated to the identification, development, and classification of nursing diagnoses.

**Nursing diagnosis** "A clinical judgment about individual, family, or community responses to actual or potential health problems/life processes. Nursing diagnoses provide the basis for selection of nursing interventions to achieve outcomes for which the nurse is accountable" (NANDA International); a name for an actual or potential health problem or life process that refers to a set of human responses; a specific class or category in a diagnostic classification system.

**Nursing outcome** Health state attributable to nursing intervention; describes resolution of a nursing diagnosis or steps toward resolution; category in a classification system that has specific clinical indicators.

**Related factors** Conditions or events having some association with a health problem.

**Risk factor** An observable sign, verbal report, or contextual attribute that is an indicator of a potential problem or risk state.

**Supporting cue** An observable sign, verbal report, or contextual attribute that serves as an indicator of more than one health problem; information that influences confidence in a diagnostic judgment; a sign or symptom; a defining characteristic, usually of one or more diagnoses.

**Taxonomy** A set of rules and procedures for classification; also used to refer to the classification system that is organized by the rules or procedures.

# Index

# INDEX

467

# INDEX

# INDEX

enhanced behavior, readiness for
  childbearing process, 407–408
  communication, 392
  coping, 416
  coping, community, 431
  coping, family, 430
  decision making, 300
  family processes, 369
  fluid balance, 133
  health management, 65
  hope, 321
  immunization status, 84
  knowledge, 286
  nutrition, 111
  organized infant behavior, 253
  parenting, 384
  power, 325
  relationships, 362
  religiosity, 458
  resilience, 425
  self-care, 216
  self-concept, 332
  sleep, 268
  spiritual well-being, 453–454
  urinary elimination, 178
environment. *See also* health
    environment
  impaired interpretation
    syndrome, 296
  relocation stress syndrome,
    359–360, 361
  support system deficit,
    436
esteem, compromised, risk for, 326
examination for health patterns, 10
  adult assessment, 15
  documentation example, 51–55
  infant and young child
    assessment, 21
excess fluid volume, 131–132
excoriation. *See* skin integrity
excretory function patterns. *See*
    elimination health pattern
exercise. *See* activity
exercise pattern. *See*
    activity–exercise health pattern
exhaustion. *See* fatigue

exogenous obesity, 106–107, 108
exposure to contaminants. *See*
    contamination

## F

failure to thrive (adult), 112–113
faith. *See* belief system; values
falls, risk for, 92–93
families
  caregiver role strain, 385–388,
    389–390
  coping, compromised, 426–427
  coping, disabled, 428–429
  coping, readiness for enhanced,
    430
  dysfunctional processes,
    365–369
  enhanced, readiness for, 369
  interrupted processes, 363–364
  parent–infant separation, 381
  parenting impairment, 370–373,
    374–375
  readiness for enhanced
    parenting, 384
  therapeutic regimen management,
    ineffective, 70
  weak parent–infant attachment,
    379–380, 381
family assessments, 21–25
fatigue, 186–187
fear, 306–307
feeding self-care deficit, 210–211
feelings. *See* emotions; self-
    perception
fetal–maternal dyad, risk for
    disturbed, 409
flow, blood. *See* blood circulation
fluid balance
  deficient volume, 128–129, 130
  electrolyte imbalance, 135
  enhanced, readiness for,
    133
  excess volume, 131–132
  risk for imbalance, 133
fluid consumption pattern. *See*
    nutritional–metabolic health
    pattern

470

# INDEX

# INDEX

# INDEX

# INDEX

# INDEX

*Continued from first page*